Preface

Haematology is a clinical subject based on an understanding of
scientific principles and laboratory investigations. Morphological
examination of blood and marrow remains the cornerstone of laboratory
haematology although this now extends into the realms of genetics,
biochemistry and immunology. This book largely comprises photographs
of blood and marrow films but is not a conventional atlas. Where
appropriate there are clinical pictures and illustrations of common
laboratory procedures. There is a brief text covering all aspects of
haematology, although emphasis is given to those areas where
microscopy is essential to the diagnosis.

It is hoped that this book will be particularly useful to those coming
to haematology for the first time, especially those faced with the
prospects of practical examinations.

We wish to acknowledge our many friends and colleagues who have
provided pathological material for photography. We would like to thank
Professor E.R. Huehns, Dr J. Richards, Dr A.H. Goldstone, Professor
J.W. Stewart, Dr K. McLennan and Dr A. Newlands, Professor S.J.
Machin and Dr M. Greaves and Dr M. Burke for contributing slides
included in this book.

We also wish to thank Ms Martine Owen for secretarial assistance.

London   D.C.L.
1996   A.P.Y.
                                                         M.J.W.

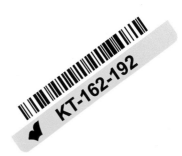
KT-162-192

Contents

1 / **The blood count / The blood film**

The blood count

The different types of blood cell are enumerated by an automated counter. Red cell volume is measured directly (mean cell volume, MCV) and serves as the basis of the classification of anaemia.

- Normocytic anaemia   MCV 78–99 fl
- Microcytic anaemia   MCV <78 fl
- Macrocytic anaemia   MCV >99 fl

The blood film

It is important to use even films made with a smooth edged spreader. The blood should be fresh, as storage in ethylenediamine tetra-acetic acid (EDTA) produces morphological artefacts. The slide should be dried and then fixed promptly in absolute methanol. Stains using eosin and methylene blue are usually used. The May-Grunwald Giemsa stain has been used routinely in this book.

The normal red cell is a little smaller than a small lymphocyte. Most red cells appear round but up to 10% may be oval. Staining is paler in the centre of the red cell reflecting its biconcave discoid shape.

The spreading action applied to the blood drop results in a thin blood film 'wedge', tapering from a thicker head to tail. In a correctly made film main white cell types should be identifiable in the thick and trail ends of the smear (Figs 1 and 2); the optimal area for red cell and white cell morphology is in the main body of the smear (Fig. 3).

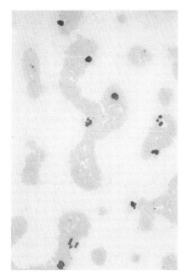

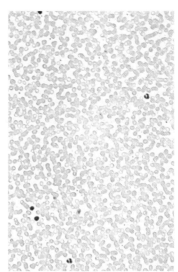

Fig. 1 Trailing edge of peripheral blood film (*low power*): incorrect area to view red cell or white cell morphology.

Fig. 2 Thick part of peripheral blood film (*low power*). Also not suitable for morphological examination.

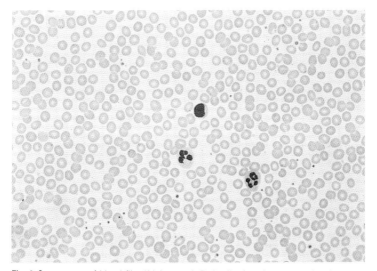

Fig. 3 Correct part of blood film (*high power*). Red cells close but not overlapping.

Neutrophils

Their diameter is a little less than twice the size of a red cell. The nucleus has 2–4 lobes made up of coarse chromatin. The cytoplasm is pale pink and contains fine violet granules (Fig. 4).

The normal adult neutrophil count is 2.0–7.5 × 10^9/l although the lower limit of normal in Negroes is $1.5 × 10^9$/l. The levels are dynamic and can rise significantly after exercise.

Aetiology of neutrophilia
- Infections, especially bacterial.
- Inflammatory conditions.
- Tissue injury.
- Myeloproliferative disorders.

Marked neutrophilia is often associated with characteristic morphological changes including a left shift (appearance of non-segmented, developmentally early neutrophils) (Figs 5 & 6), toxic granulation (Fig. 7), toxic vacuolation (usually indicative of sepsis) and Dohle bodies.

Aetiology of neutropenia
- Occasional bacterial infections such as typhoid, and overwhelming sepsis.
- HIV infection.
- Aplastic anaemia.
- Marrow infiltration.
- Megaloblastic anaemia.
- Hypersplenism.
- Immune destruction.
- Drugs (immune and non-immune).

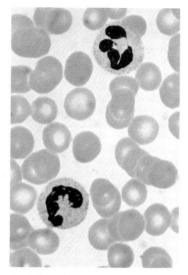

Fig. 4 Normal neutrophils (granulocytes).

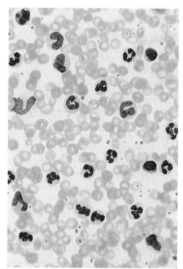

Fig. 5 Neutrophilia with mature polymorphs.

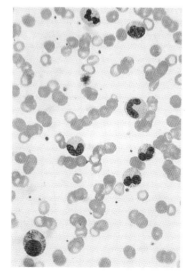

Fig. 6 Neutrophilia with poorly segmented forms (left shift) indicating release of bone marrow stores.

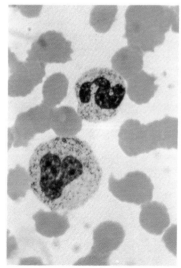

Fig. 7 Increased 'toxic granulation' of the neutrophils in a patient with sepsis.

Eosinophils

Similar in size to the neutrophil but usually only two lobes to the nucleus. The cytoplasm is filled with large eosinophilic granules (Fig. 8). The normal count is $<0.4 \times 10^9/l$.

Aetiology of eosinophilia
- Allergic conditions including drugs.
- Parasitic infections.
- Occasional bacterial infections.
- Skin diseases.
- Inflammatory disorders of the gut.
- Pulmonary eosinophilia.
- Hodgkin's disease and other haematological malignancies.
- Langerhan's cell histiocytoses.

Hypereosinophilic syndrome
This is defined as persistent elevation of the eosinophil count ($>1.5 \times 10^9/l$) (Fig. 9) of uncertain cause for more than 6 months. The patients are typically unwell, febrile and often have damage to the lungs and heart. Treatment is initially with steroids and then with cytotoxic drugs (e.g. hydroxyurea) if these fail.

Basophils

Similar size to neutrophils with a nucleus consisting of 2–3 lobes. Cytoplasm contains large purple/black granules (Fig. 10). Normal count $<0.1 \times 10^9/l$, i.e. a rare cell.

Aetiology of basophilia
- Myeloproliferative disorders especially chronic myeloid leukaemia.
- Occasionally in chronic infections.
- Severe hypothyroidism.

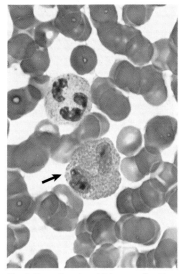

Fig. 8 Normal eosinophil (*arrowed*) with normal neutrophil.

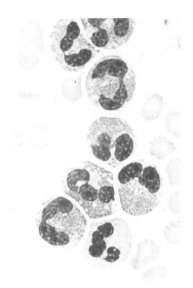

Fig. 9 Eosinophils from a case of hypereosinophilic syndrome.

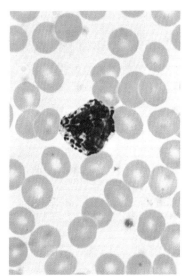

Fig. 10 A basophil. These are infrequent cells in normal blood smears.

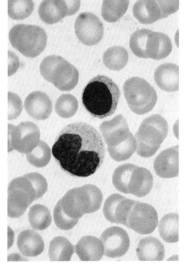

Fig. 11 Normal monocyte compared to a lymphocyte.

Monocytes

Monocytes are large cells. The nucleus is often irregular or kidney shaped. The cytoplasm is typically sky-blue in colour and may contain vacuoles or scanty fine red granules (Fig. 11, p. 6).

Aetiology of monocytosis
- Convalescence from many acute infections.
- Some chronic bacterial infections.
- Viral infections, especially children.
- Collagen vascular diseases.
- Preleukaemia and monocytic leukaemia.

Lymphocytes

The lymphocyte population is heterogeneous (Figs 12, 13 & 14). The small lymphocyte has a dense chromatin pattern and has little cytoplasm. Larger lymphocytes have more cytoplasm and the nucleus may be irregular. The cytoplasm may contain reddish granules. The normal adult count is $1.5-4.0 \times 10^9/l$. About 70% of lymphocytes in the blood are T cells (approximately two-thirds CD4 and one-third CD8), 5–10% are B cells and the remainder are non-T non-B cells.

Aetiology of lymphocytosis
- Infections.
- Malignant lymphoproliferative disorders.
- Autoimmune disorders.

Aetiology of lymphopenia
- Congenital immune deficiency.
- Following cytotoxic drugs, radiography or steroid administration.
- Hodgkin's disease and some other lymphomas.
- Severe aplastic anaemia.
- Some infections.
- Postoperative.
- Autoimmune disorders.

Platelets

Platelets are less than one-third the diameter of a red cell. They are round or oval and have an irregular outline. They are pale blue with reddish granules and no nucleus. The causes of thrombocytosis and thrombocytopenia are discussed on pages 127–131.

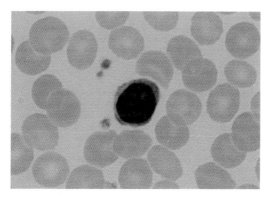

Fig. 12 Small lymphocyte (normal film).

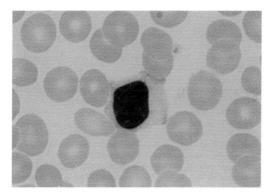

Fig. 13 Large lymphocyte (normal film).

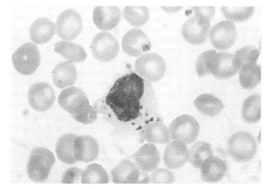

Fig. 14 Lymphocyte with azurophil granules (normal film).

2 / Normal bone marrow

The bone marrow is obtained by 'needle aspiration' or 'core biopsy'. The marrow is the site of postnatal haemopoiesis and the quantity and quality of haemopoietic precursor cells can be assessed from the marrow films. Cellularity can be estimated from inspection of the marrow fragments at low power (Fig. 15). Between 25% and 75% of the fragment volume should consist of marrow cells, the remainder being fat cells. Cellularity is better determined from sections of a large core biopsy (Fig. 16). As in the blood, all cell lines should be studied in turn. It is convenient to first look for megakaryocytes as these are best seen at low power. Megakaryocytes often segregate at the edges and trails of the film (Fig. 17).

Platelet series

Megakaryoblast
↓
Megakaryocytes
↓
Platelets

Megakaryoblasts are very rare cells and not usually identified. Megakaryocytes are very large cells with great variation in size. The nucleus is polyploid with 4–16 lobules. The cytoplasm is blue/grey with reddish granules (Fig. 18).

The regulation of platelet production is partly controlled by a series of haemopoietic growth factors especially thrombopoietin.

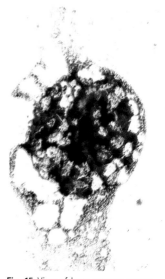

Fig. 15 View of bone marrow smear showing normocellular fragment (*low power*).

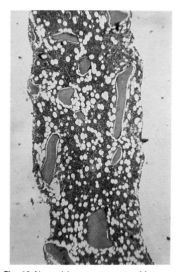

Fig. 16 Normal bone marrow trephine biopsy in a young adult (*low power*).

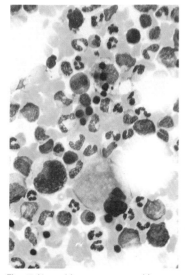

Fig. 17 Normal bone marrow trephine biopsy (*med. power*) showing megakaryocyte.

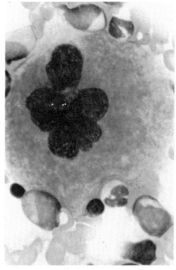

Fig. 18 Megakaryocyte on bone marrow smear (*high power*).

Red cell series

Proerythroblast
↓
Early normoblast
↓
Intermediate normoblast
↓
Late normoblast
↓
Red cell

The proerythroblast is a large cell with a high nuclear to cytoplasmic ratio. The nucleus has a coarse interwoven appearance and may contain up to 5 nucleoli. The cytoplasm is deep blue although there is often a perinuclear pale zone (Fig. 19). With maturation the nucleus becomes smaller and the chromatin more condensed. The cells also become smaller but the cytoplasmic proportion increases. The cytoplasm changes from blue to pink as haemoglobin accumulates (Figs 20 & 21).

A number of growth factors including stem cell factor and interleukin 3 (IL-3) affect the proliferation of primitive red cells. The later stages of erythropoiesis are regulated by erythropoietin which is produced by the peritubular cells in the kidney in response to tissue hypoxia.

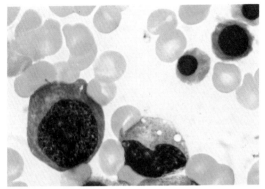

Fig. 19 Proerythroblast.

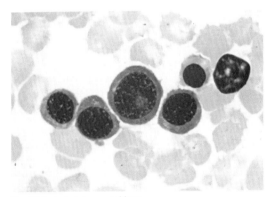

Fig. 20 Early to late normoblasts.

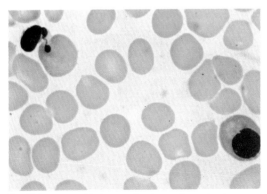

Fig. 21 Late normoblasts: one showing nuclear extrusion.

Granulocyte cell series

Myeloblast
↓
Promyelocyte
↓
Myelocyte
↓
Metamyelocyte
↓
Granulocyte

The myeloblast varies in size from just a little larger than a red cell to two or three times this size. There is a high nuclear to cytoplasmic ratio. The nucleus has a fine chromatin pattern with 2–4 nucleoli. The cytoplasm is blue in colour and contains no granules (Figs. 22, 23). The promyelocyte is a larger cell than the myeloblast with more cytoplasm which now contains primary granules. Nucleoli are still apparent in the nucleus. With progressive maturation, the cells become smaller, the nucleolus disappears, the nucleus becomes more condensed, oval, then horseshoe shaped and finally segmented (Figs. 22, 23). Small secondary granules appear in the cytoplasm replacing the larger primary granules. The vast majority of the granulocyte series are of the neutrophil lineage.

Production of neutrophils is predominantly regulated by granulocyte colony stimulating factor (G-CSF) the serum levels of which rise in response to neutropenia and infection. Monocyte colony stimulating factor is involved in the production of monocytes and their transition to tissue macrophages. The production of eosinophils is regulated by granulocyte-macrophage colony stimulating factor (GM-CSF) and interleukin 5 (IL-5).

Lymphocyte series

In adults lymphocytes are a minor population in the bone marrow (5–20%). Precursor lymphoblasts are rare cells although they may be more prominent in children.

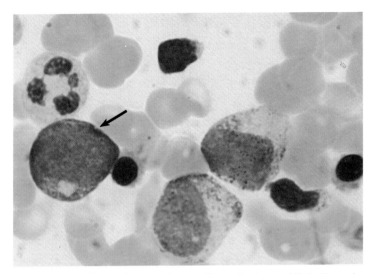

Fig. 22 Myeloblast (*arrowed*), two myelocytes with prominant azurophilic (red) granules and a mature neutrophil.

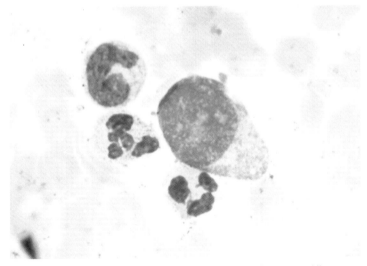

Fig. 23 Large myeloblast with two segmented and one 'band' form neutrophil.

3 / Classification of anaemia

From a pathophysiological viewpoint anaemia can be considered as due to either defective red blood cell production or excessive erythrocyte loss. In the modern clinical setting anaemia is initially characterized by inspection of the printout from an automated haemoglobin and cell counter. The haemoglobin and red cell size (MCV) are measured directly. The MCV can later be confirmed on microscopy.

Important information about the aetiology of anaemia is often obtained from the history and examination. The white blood cell count, platelet count, reticulocyte count and blood film all produce further relevant information.

Normocytic anaemia (MCV 78–99fl) (Fig. 24)
- Following blood loss.
- Haemolysis.
- Chronic disease.
- Combined iron and folate deficiency.

May be microcytic if secondary iron deficiency develops; mildly macrocytic if a reticulocytosis

Microcytic anaemia (MCV <78fl)
- Iron deficiency (Fig. 25).
- Thalassaemia.
- Chronic disease.
- Sideroblastic anaemia.

Macrocytic anaemia (MCV >99fl)
- Megaloblastic (Fig. 26).
- Non-megaloblastic.

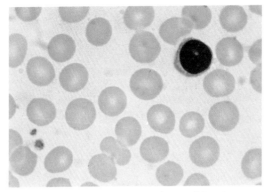

Fig. 24 Normocytic red cells compared to small lymphocyte.

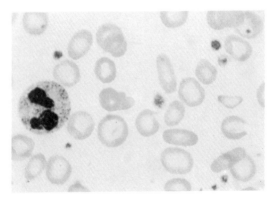

Fig. 25 Microcytic and hypochromic blood film.

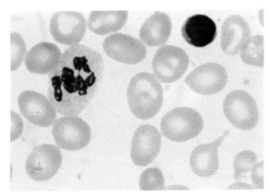

Fig. 26 Macrocytic blood film.

4 / Iron deficiency

Incidence   Over 10% of many Western urban populations are
iron deficient though not all are anaemic. In many
other parts of the world the incidence is still higher.
Iron deficiency is particularly common in women of
child bearing age.

Aetiology   • *Poor diet.*
• *Malabsorption of iron:*
  —following gastric surgery (rapid transit)
  —achlorhydria—HCl is required for the absorption
   of ferric salts
  —Coeliac disease/tropical sprue.
• *Blood loss.* This may be via heavy menstruation, or
  bleeding from the gut or renal tract.
• *Other rare causes* include:
  —intravascular haemolysis
  —pulmonary siderosis.

Clinical features   • General features of anaemia, including dyspnoea on
  effort, weakness, dizziness and headaches.
• Angular stomatitis and atrophic glossitis.
• Brittle spoon-shaped nails (koilonychia) (Fig. 27).
• Brittle sparse hair.
• Pruritis vulvae.
• Pica in children.
• Rarely a posterior cricoid web may develop
  (Plummer-Vinson syndrome) (Fig. 28).

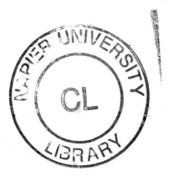

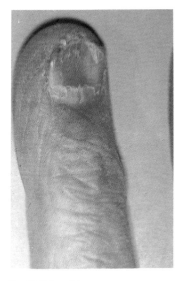

Fig. 27 Koilonychia.

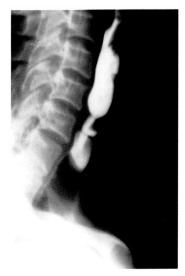

Fig. 28 Posterior cricoid web in severe iron deficiency: a rare feature.

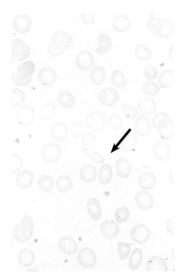

Fig. 29 Iron deficiency blood film showing microcytosis, hypochromia, anisocytosis, poikilocytosis and characteristic pencil cell (*arrowed*).

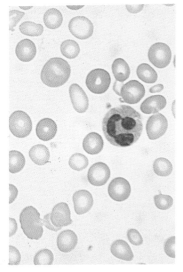

Fig. 30 Dimorphic blood film. Microcytic/hypochromic red cells with a population of normochromic cells.

Investigations   Microcytosis (MCV <78fl) appears first and progresses as anaemia develops. Red cells show microcytosis, hypochromia, anisocytosis (variation in size) and poikilocytosis (variation in shape). Pencil cells are characteristic (Fig. 29, p. 18). The leukocyte count and platelet count are usually normal.

The marrow is cellular. Erythropoiesis is normoblastic. Myelopoiesis and megakaryocytes are normal. Iron staining of marrow particles reveals an absence of iron.

Serum iron is low (normal range 10–30 μmol/1). Total iron binding capacity (TIBC) is high normal or raised (normal range 40–70 μmol/1). The % saturation (serum/iron TIBC) is usually <10%. The serum ferritin is reduced: usually <10 μg/dl, although it may be misleadingly higher if there is a coexistent inflammatory disorder.

Once iron deficiency is established the underlying cause must be established by thorough history taking, physical examination, and relevant further investigations.

Treatment   **Oral iron**. Oral iron is given to correct the anaemia (Fig. 30, p. 18) and then replete the body stores (3–6 months) (Figs 31 & 32). Ferrous sulphate 200 mg t.d.s. is cheap and effective though the dose must be reduced in occasional patients who experience side-effects.

Parenteral iron. This should only be used if oral iron cannot be tolerated, or if negative iron balance persists. Parenteral iron can be given as a course of intramuscular injections or rarely as an intravenous iron infusion. The latter procedure is hazardous.

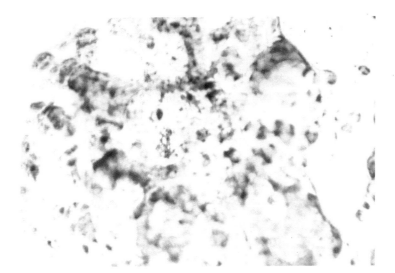

Fig. 31 Normal marrow fragment showing iron particles staining with Prussian Blue.

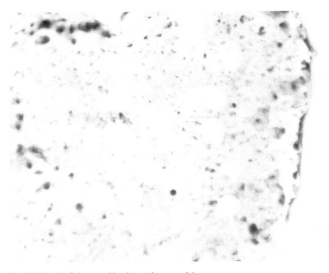

Fig. 32 Iron deficiency with absent iron particles.

5 / Megaloblastic anaemias

This group of disorders is characterized by reduced DNA synthesis (not just in red cell series) associated with pathognomonic morphological changes in the blood and marrow (Fig. 33 & Figs 36–39, p. 24).

Aetiology
- *Folate deficiency.*
- *B12 deficiency.*
- *Some cytotoxic drugs*, e.g. methotrexate, cytosine arabinoside.
- *Rare causes* including certain inborn errors of metabolism.

Causes of B12 deficiency
- Malabsorption (absorbed mainly in terminal ileum):
  —'pernicious anaemia' of immune origin leading to failure of intrinsic factor production (Figs 34 & 35).
  —intrinsic factor deficiency secondary to surgery
  —terminal ileal disease (site of B12 absorption)
  —competitive parasites, esp. bacterial overgrowth with 'blind loops'
  —pancreatic failure
  —occasional drugs.
- Nutritional deficiency in vegans and alcoholics.

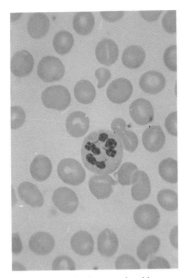

Fig. 33 Megaloblastic anaemia with multisegmented neutrophil.

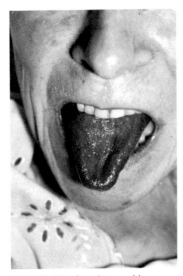

Fig. 34 Red 'beef steak tongue' in pernicious anaemia.

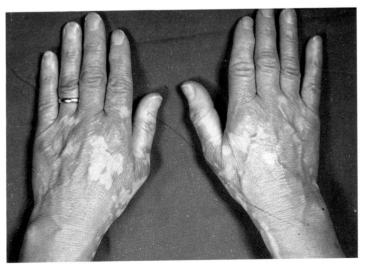

Fig. 35 Loss of pigment (vitiligo) in megaloblastic anaemia.

Causes of folate deficiency

- Nutritional deficiency. Especially common at the extremes of age and in alcoholics.
- Malabsorption (absorbed mainly in upper jejunum):
  —gastrectomy
  —coeliac disease/tropical sprue
  —extensive Crohn's disease
  —phenytoin (interferes with absorption).
- Increased requirements, including pregnancy, lactation, rapid growth, haemolysis, malignancies and repeated dialysis.
- Defective folate utilization seen with antifolate drugs, some anticonvulsants and alcohol.

Clinical features of megaloblastic anaemia

Very insidious onset of anaemia. Hb may be as low as 2 g/dl at presentation. Anorexia and glossitis are common. There may be fevers, recurrent infections and petechiae in severe cases. Subacute combined degeneration of the cord can occur with B12 deficiency.

Investigations

Low Hb with a raised MCV. In the early stages macrocytosis appears before the anaemia. The red cells show anisocytosis, poikilocytosis and may contain inclusion bodies. The neutrophil count is often reduced and multisegmented neutrophils are characteristic (Fig. 33, p. 22). The platelet count is often reduced.

The marrow is hypercellular with megaloblastic changes in both the red and white cell series (Figs 36–39).

Treatment

- Treat any underlying cause if possible.
- Replace deficient haematinic. B12 is given by i.m. injections. After replacing stores it is usual to give 1000 μg hydroxycobalamin every 3 months. Folate should not be given in B12 deficiency as it may exacerbate the neurological condition. Folate is usually given orally even in malabsorption.

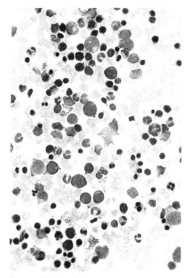

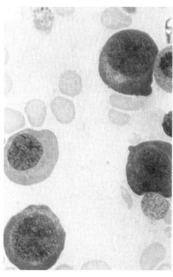

Fig. 36 Marrow fragments in megaloblastic anaemia (*low power*) showing erythroid hypercellularity.

Fig. 37 Megaloblasts—nuclear fenestration.

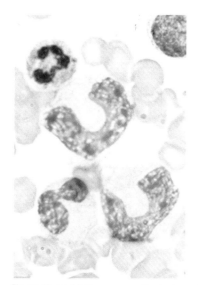

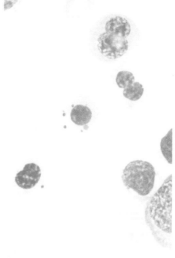

Fig. 38 Megaloblastic marrow with giant metamyelocytes.

Fig. 39 Nuclear abnormalities in megaloblasts including polar bodies.

6 / Aplastic anaemia

There is depression of the blood elements in association with reduced haemopoietic tissue in the marrow.

Aetiology
- *Congenital*
  The commonest of these disorders is Fanconi's anaemia. This is an autosomal recessive disease usually presenting at 4–7 years. Bony and renal abnormalities are common. The erythrocyte sedimentation rate (ESR) is usually high, the marrow may appear megaloblastic and HbF is often high.
- *Chronic acquired:*
  —idiopathic
  —drugs, chemicals or irradiation
  —associated with some infections especially viral hepatitis
  —associated with paroxysmal nocturnal haemoglobinuria
  —other rare associations including pregnancy.
- *Acute transient*
  Usually due to infections but can be any of the above acquired causes.

Clinical features
Insidious onset of symptoms due to anaemia, bleeding and infections (Fig. 40).

Investigations
Anaemia which may be normocytic or mildly macrocytic.

—absolute reticulocytopenia.
—absolute granulocytopenia.
—monocytopenia is usual.
—platelets decreased.

Marrow shows abundant fat spaces and few haemopoietic cells (Figs 41 & 42).

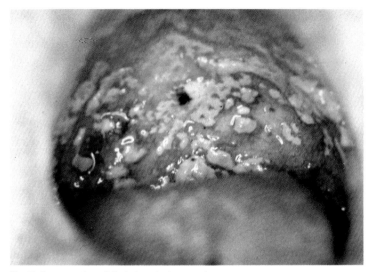

Fig. 40 Severe oral candidiasis in aplastic anaemia.

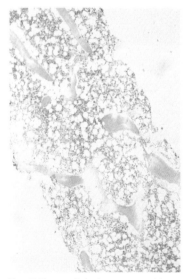

Fig. 41 Normocellular bone marrow biopsy (*low power*).

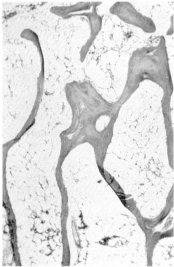

Fig. 42 Severely hypoplastic marrow biopsy. Compare to Figure 41.

Treatment
- *Supportive care.* Infection is the most likely cause of death in aplastic anaemia and must be treated early and aggressively. Multiple swabs and cultures should be sent before starting broad-spectrum antibiotics. Red cell and platelet support must be given when required.
- *Attempts to stimulate the marrow:*
  —Androgens are often given, but benefit, if any, tends to be small.
  —Haemopoietic growth factors such as G-CSF may increase the neutrophil count but are mostly effective in mild cases only.
  —Immunosuppressive high-dose steroids and anti-lymphocyte globulin may be partly effective.
- *Bone marrow transplantation (BMT).* Severe disease in those <40 years, especially children, is probably best treated by BMT if there is a matched sibling donor available.

Pure red cell aplasia (PRCA)

Acute
This is usually a self-limiting episode in patients with congenital haemolytic anaemias. It is due to a parvovirus infection (Fifth's disease).

Chronic

Congenital (Diamond Blackfan syndrome).
Usually inherited but mode uncertain. It is often associated with other minor congenital abnormalities. Anaemia usually begins in the first few days of life but may be delayed for several years. Very few normoblasts are seen in the marrow. The HbF is usually raised. Many patients respond to steroids and others require transfusion.

Acquired. Often associated with a thymoma or an established autoimmune disease (Figs 44 & 45).

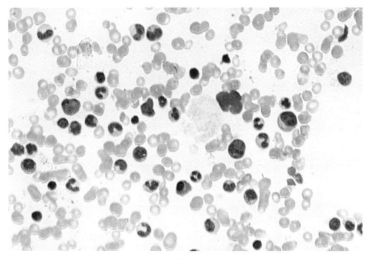

Fig. 43 Bone marrow film showing red cell hypoplasia.

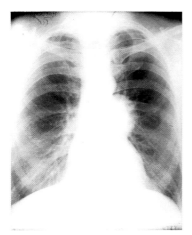

Fig. 44 CXR (*PA*) showing large thymoma associated with PRCA.

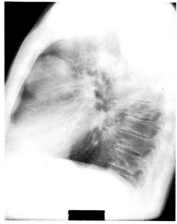

Fig. 45 CXR (*lateral*) localising to thymoma, anterior mediastinum.

7 / General features of haemolytic anaemia

Clinical features
- Features of anaemia.
- Mild jaundice.
- Variable degrees of splenomegaly.
- Occasional leg ulcers in chronic cases (Fig. 46).
- Occasional biliary colic in chronic cases (pigment gallstones).

Investigations *Evidence of red cell destruction.*

- Reduced Hb. MCV may be normal or increased.
- Reticulocytosis (Fig. 47).
- The blood film may show abnormal red cells, e.g. sickle cells, spherocytes.
- Raised serum Hb (intravascular haemolysis) (Fig. 48). Haemoglobinuria (intravascular haemolysis; Fig. 54, p. 34) and haemosiderinuria in chronic cases (Fig. 55, p. 34).
- Raised bilirubin: unconjugated, indirect van den Bergh reaction.
- Marrow erythroid hyperplasia (Fig. 49).
- In chronic haemolysis in childhood, expanded marrow cavities lead to bossing of the skull (Fig. 59, p. 38).

Aetiology
The potential causes of haemolysis are enormous. Careful history, examination and study of the peripheral blood film provide essential clues in most cases.

The direct antiglobulin test (DAT) to detect the presence of antibody on the red cells (immune haemolysis) is the next step (Fig. 71, p. 46).

In cases of DAT-negative haemolysis with no obvious clues from the history, examination or blood film, an empirical approach to investigations must be adopted, bearing in mind which disorders are relatively common, e.g. G6PD deficiency.

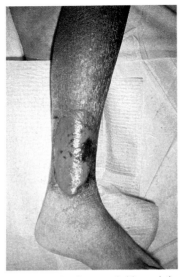

Fig. 46 Leg ulcer in congenital haemolytic anaemia.

Fig. 47 Reticulocytosis shown using supravital staining (New Methylene Blue).

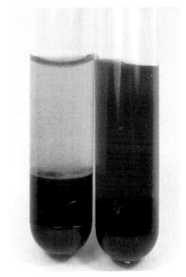

Fig. 48 Plasma containing free haemoglobin in severe intravascular haemolysis (*right*).

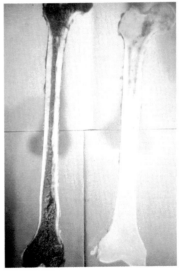

Fig. 49 Red marrow extension in congenital haemolysis (*left*) contrasted with an aplastic anaemia marrow (*right*).

8 / **Disorders of the red cell membrane**

Spherocytosis Hereditary spherocytosis (HS) is an inherited condition (usually autosomal dominant) in which the red cells are more rigid and fragile than normal. They are spherocytic in shape appearing small and deeply stained on blood smears (Fig. 50), and have a high osmotic fragility. The spleen is usually palpable. Any anaemia is usually mild, but the Hb may fall considerably with intercurrent infections (aplastic crises) or during periods of increased splenic sequestration (haemolytic crises).

Jaundice is usually mild, if detectable, but may rarely be a cause of kernicterus.

Splenectomy improves the haemolysis and is performed if indicated, preferably after childhood. Penicillin should be given to splenectomized patients.

Spherocytes are also seen in some immune-mediated haemolytic anaemias.

Elliptocytosis Hereditary elliptocytosis is an inherited condition (usually autosomal dominant) in which the majority of cells have an elliptical shape (Fig. 51). The osmotic fragility is normal.

Most affected individuals are asymptomatic, though mild anaemia, jaundice, splenomegaly and leg ulcers can occur.

Elliptocytes can also occur in iron deficiency and megaloblastic anaemia.

Stomatocytosis Stomatocytosis (mouth like) may be inherited or occur in a variety of acquired disorders including thalassaemia, liver disease and alcoholism (Fig. 52).

Acanthocytosis This may be inherited (autosomal recessive) in
('Burr cells') association with retinitis pigmentosa, diffuse neurological deficits, and aβ-lipoproteinaemia. Acanthocytes are also seen in renal failure, cirrhosis, microangiopathic haemolytic anaemia, and as an artifact in blood stored in EDTA (Fig. 53).

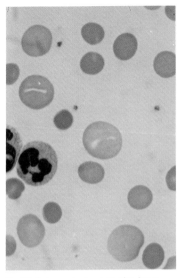

Fig. 50 Spherocytosis—note also large polychromatic (increased RNA) red cells.

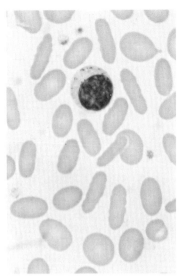

Fig. 51 Elliptocytosis.

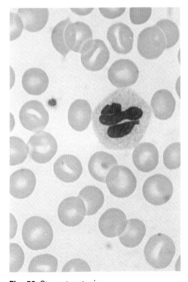

Fig. 52 Stomatocytosis.

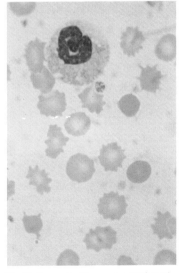

Fig. 53 Burr cells. These were artefactual due to storage in EDTA Note degenerate leucocyte.

Paroxysmal nocturnal haemoglobinuria

In paroxysmal nocturnal haemoglobinuria (PNH) there is a clone of abnormal haemopoietic stem cells in which there is a deficiency of molecules normally anchored to the membrane by phosphatidyl inositol linkages. The gene responsible for PNH is carried on the X chromosome and both males and females may be affected. The red cell membranes are abnormally sensitive to complement.

Clinical features
- Mild anaemia of gradual onset.
- Mild jaundice.
- Haemoglobinuria especially after sleeping.
- Hepatosplenomegaly common.
- Frequent urinary tract infections.
- Bleeding problems may occur.
- Thromboses may occur. These are often at unusual sites, e.g. hepatic vein.
- Aplastic anaemia. This may follow classical PNH; in other cases it is the first manifestation of PNH.

Investigations
- There is usually anaemia and often neutropenia and thrombocytopenia.
- Iron deficiency is common.
- Haemoglobin and haemosiderin may be found in the urine (Figs 54 & 55).
- The neutrophil alkaline phosphatase (NAP) score is low. There is increased sensitivity of the red cells to lysis in acidified serum (Ham's test; Fig. 56).
- Diagnosis can also be made by immunophenotypic demonstration of low/absent membrane antigens, e.g. CD59 on red cells and CD67 on granulocytes.

Treatment
- Supportive.
- Splenectomy is hazardous.

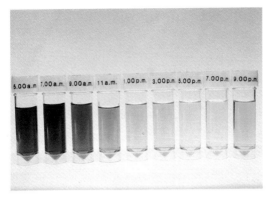

Fig. 54 Serial urines in a patient with PNH.

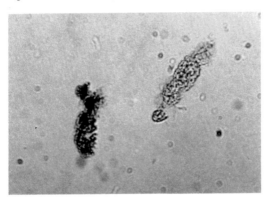

Fig. 55 Haemosiderin in urinary tract cells (urine deposit, Perl's stain).

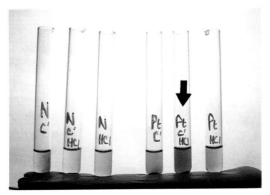

Fig. 56 Increased red cell lysis in acidified serum (Ham's test).

9 / Red cell enzyme defects

G6PD deficiency

Glucose 6 phosphate dehydrogenase (G6PD) deficiency affects approximately 100 million individuals. It is common in Africa, around the Mediterranean and in the Orient. It is X-linked.

Clinical features
- Intermittent haemolysis. This may be caused by drugs (e.g. sulphonamides, some antimalarials), fava beans, infections or other acute illnesses. In Negroes the disease is self-limiting as reticulocytes have normal enzyme activity; this is not the case in Mediterranean and Oriental varieties.
- Chronic haemolytic anaemia.
- Neonatal jaundice.

Investigations
There is anaemia and reticulocytes and Heinz bodies are seen on the reticulocyte stain (Fig. 57).

Diagnosis
There is a simple screening test for G6PD deficiency but care must be taken in Negroes with a reticulocytosis to avoid false negative results. G6PD can also be measured spectrophotometrically (Fig. 58) and the enzyme detected on electrophoretic gels.

Treatment
This is primarily the avoidance of factors that precipitate haemolysis. Transfusion may be necessary in severe cases.

PK deficiency

Pyruvate kinase (PK) deficiency is an autosomal recessive condition in which there may be moderate or even severe haemolytic anaemia.

Other enzyme deficiencies

Many other enzyme deficiencies can cause haemolysis. These are all rare.

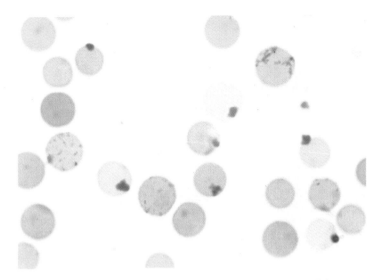

Fig. 57 Heinz bodies—note their location in proximity to the membrane and the associated reticulocytes present.

Generation of NADPH from NADP

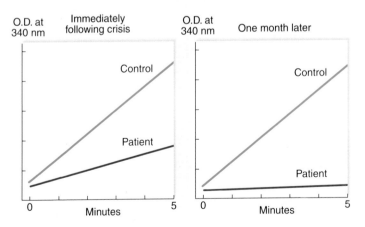

Fig. 58 Diagram of G6PD determinations. Note significant activity in this Negro patient during acute haemolysis (reticulocytes).

10 / Thalassaemias

Aetiology These are inherited disorders in which there is an abnormality of one or more of the globin genes leading to reduced globin protein production. There is therefore an imbalance of β:α globin chain synthesis leading to globin chain precipitation, ineffective erythropoiesis and haemolysis. Thalassaemia is widespread around the Mediterranean, in Africa, in the Middle East and the Far East.

Clinical syndromes of the β thalassaemias

Thalassaemia major (disease)
This occurs when both β genes are thalassaemic. Anaemia develops at about 2 months of age (after HbF→HbA switch). Untreated there is failure to thrive and physical retardation. The child develops bossing of the skull (Fig. 59), 'mongoloid' facies and hepatosplenomegaly. Death usually occurs in childhood if untreated.

Thalassaemia minor (trait)
Affected individuals have only one affected β gene. Anaemia is either not present or very mild.

Thalassaemia intermedia
This is a heterogenous group of disorders in which both β genes and sometimes one or more α genes are affected but the disease process is relatively mild with no transfusion requirement and little physical retardation.

Investigations The Hb is variably reduced. The red cells are invariably microcytic in all types of the disorder. In the disease state target cells, stippled cells and nucleated red cells are seen in the blood (Figs 60 & 61). In β thalassaemia trait HbF is usually normal and HbA_2 is slightly raised (5%). In disease, there is increased HbF and HbA_2. HbA may be absent (homozygous β° thalassaemia).

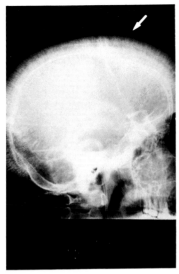

Fig. 59 Thalassaemic skull showing intramedullary expansion with bossing and 'hair on end' appearance (*arrowed*).

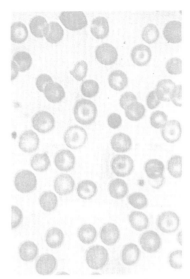

Fig. 60 Target cells in thalassaemia.

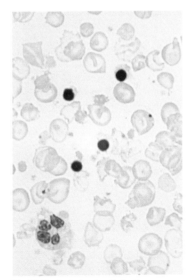

Fig. 61 Nucleated red cells in the peripheral blood in a case of thalassaemia intermedia.

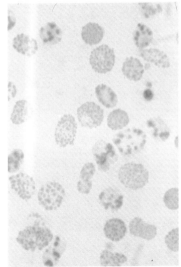

Fig. 62 HbH disease. HbH bodies are similar to Heinz bodies but multiple and often with 'golf ball' distribution within red cell.

*Clinical
syndromes of the
α thalassaemias*

Silent α thalassaemia
Only one of the genes is affected and a slight
reduction in the MCV is the only abnormality.

Thalassaemia trait
Two or three α genes are affected and individuals
may be asymptomatic or mildly anaemic.

Hb Bart's hydrops fetalis
All four α genes are involved, leading to inadequate
HbF production with intrauterine death.

Investigations

The MCV is reduced and HbH (β_4 tetramers
inclusion bodies) may be seen in the red cells
(Fig. 62, p. 38). Electrophoresis shows the presence
of HbH (not in silent form) and there may be a small
amount of Hb Barts (γ_4), especially at birth. HbA_2 is
not raised. In hydrops fetalis there is no HbA, HbA_2
or HbF; only Hb Barts and some embryonic
haemoglobins.

Treatment

In α and β thalassaemia trait problems usually only
arise with infections or during pregnancy. Folic acid is
usually given throughout pregnancy. It is important to
prevent patients being given iron supplements because
of the low MCV.

In β thalassaemia disease a high transfusion regimen
with continuous subcutaneous desferrioxamine is given
to prevent iron overload (Figs 63 & 64). Splenectomy
is required if the transfusion requirement increases.

All women with a low MCV at an antenatal
booking clinic should be screened for thalassaemia
trait; so also should the father if the mother has the
trait. Prenatal diagnosis is performed at approximately
12 weeks gestation by molecular analysis of chorionic
villus samples.

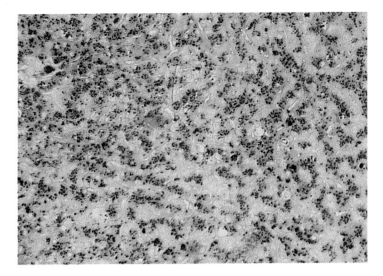

Fig. 63 Increased hepatic iron in β-thalassaemia major (*low power*).

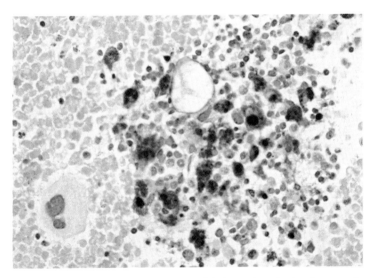

Fig. 64 Increased bone marrow macrophage in β-thalassaemia major (*medium power*).

11 / Sickle cell disease (HbS)

Aetiology   A single base mutation on the β-globin gene leads to the substitution of valine for glutamine at the 6th amino acid position of the β-globin chain. High levels of deoxygenated sickle Hb form reversible fibrils leading to sickling of the red cells.

Clinical features   The heterozygous state (trait) is usually asymptomatic, although problems may arise with anaesthesia (hypoxia). There is no anaemia. Sickle cell disease usually presents after 6 months of age, as HbF recedes. There are:

- Vaso-occlusive crises with associated infarct pain affecting particularly the bones, joints and abdominal organs. Aseptic femoral necrosis, dactylitis (Fig. 65), renal damage, priapism and retinopathy all may occur.
- Anaemia may be due to haemolysis, 'aplastic crises' precipitated by parvovirus infection, folate deficiency and sequestration crises in the liver or spleen.
- Splenomegaly is common in childhood but disappears as the spleen is infarcted.
- Leg ulceration (Fig. 66).

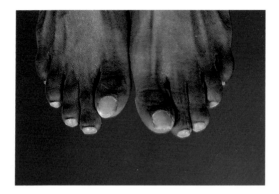

Fig. 65 Dactylitis showing shortened big toe.

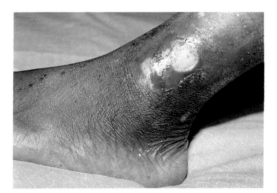

Fig. 66 Leg ulcers in sickle disease.

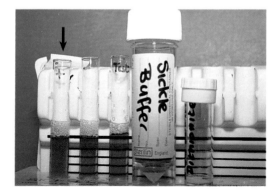

Fig. 67 Sickle screening test—positive (turbid; arrowed) and negative (clear) controls with a negative test result.

Investigations   The blood appears normal in the trait, although the sickle screening test is positive (Fig. 67, p. 42). In the disease there is mild to moderate normocytic anaemia, with reticulocytes and sickle cells on the peripheral blood film (Fig. 68). Hb electrophoresis shows HbS and no HbA (Fig. 70).

Management
- Prevention; patients with SS should avoid dehydration, hypoxia, acidosis or cold. Infections should be treated promptly.
- Crises are treated by analgesia, hydration and correction of any precipitating factors.
- A hypertransfusion regimen may be indicated in severely affected individuals.
- Bone marrow transplantation may be justified in severely affected children, particularly those who have had cerebrovascular incidents.

Other sickling disorders

Sickle thalassaemia
Sickling can arise when there is 'sickle trait' in association with β thalassaemia.

Haemoglobin C
Homozygotes may have mild sickling episodes, and splenomegaly. HbS/C (Fig. 69) is renowned for ocular complications.

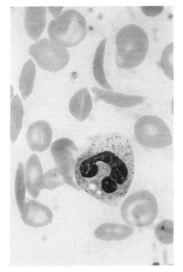

Fig. 68 Sickle cells.

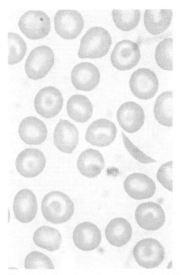

Fig. 69 Sickle cells and target cells in HbS/C disease.

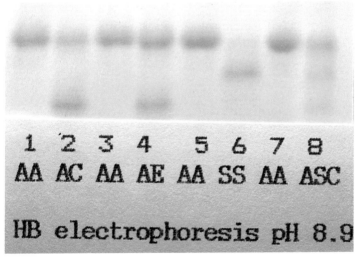

Fig. 70 Mobility of common haemoglobins by cellulose acetate electrophoresis at pH 8.9.

12 / Immune haemolytic anaemia (IHA)

Immune haemolytic anaemias (IHAs) are characterized by a positive direct antiglobulin test (Fig. 71). Spherocytes are frequently seen on the blood film (Fig. 72). IHAs are classified as:

Warm antibody type
Usually IgG antibodies which react best at 37°C.

- Primary idiopathic.
- Secondary to other autoimmune diseases, lymphoproliferative disorders and some infections.

The onset of haemolysis is usually gradual and is often chronic.

Treatment consists of transfusions if necessary, steroids and splenectomy if steroids fail.

Azathiaprine may also be useful in some cases.

Cold antibody type
Exposure to cold results in red cell agglutination with subsequent haemolysis. This is usually due to IgM antibodies.

- Idiopathic cold haemagglutinin disease (CHAD).
- CHAD secondary to autoimmune disorders, lymphoproliferative disorders and *Mycoplasma pneumoniae* infections.

CHAD can give rise to acute episodes of haemolysis or to chronic mild anaemia. Cold often causes Raynaud's syndrome. Red cell agglutinates are seen on the blood film (Fig. 73). In mild cases avoidance of cold is all that is necessary. In severe cases chlorambucil or cyclophosphamide may help.

Associated with drugs
This may be due to drugs acting as haptens absorbed on to red cells, drug-antibody immune complexes absorbed on to red cells or to stimulation of antibodies to pre-existing red cell antigens.

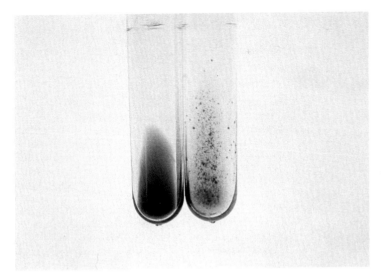

Fig. 71 Positive direct antiglobin test (DAT) (*right*).

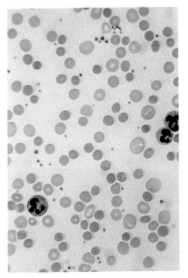

Fig. 72 Spherocytes in autoimmune haemolytic anaemia (AIHA).

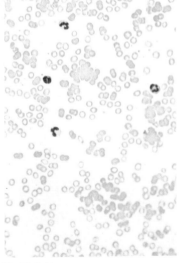

Fig. 73 Cold aggregates.

Transfusion reactions

Haemolytic disease of the newborn (HDN)

Antigen-negative mothers bearing an antigen-positive child are frequently immunized by fetal cells at birth. The number of fetal red cells that enter the maternal circulation can be estimated with the Kleihauer test (Fig. 74). In subsequent pregnancies with an antigen-positive fetus IgG antibodies are formed which cross the placenta and cause haemolysis in the fetus. Most cases of immune HDN are due to antibodies to the rhesus D antigen. Nearly 15% of births are to rhesus D-negative mothers with a D^+ father and 75% of these children will be D^+.

Clinical features There is anaemia in the affected fetus or child associated with nucleated red blood cells in the neonate's blood (Fig. 75). At birth the child is not severely jaundiced because of the placental clearance system, but jaundice may worsen rapidly and produce kernicterus if not treated promptly. In its severest form, there is cardiac failure, hepatosplenomegaly, and intrauterine death (hydrops fetalis).

Diagnosis The blood group of the mother is routinely assessed, and the father is also tested if the mother is D negative. A previous history of pregnancies, previously affected infants, abortions and blood transfusions (possible sensitization) is essential. During the pregnancy antibodies can be measured in the maternal serum, and bilirubin can be measured in the amniotic fluid to assess the severity of the haemolysis. At birth the degree of anaemia is the best guide to the severity.

Treatment
- In severe cases intrauterine transfusion must be given. Transfused cells must be compatible with the mother's serum.
- Exchange transfusion may be required soon after birth to prevent kernicterus. Fresh blood should be used.
- Phototherapy may augment bilirubin breakdown and avoid the necessity of exchange transfusion in mild cases (Fig. 76).

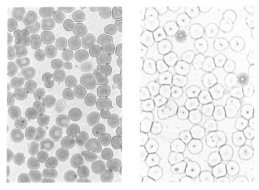

Fig. 74 Kleihauer test: HbF is resistant to acid elution and stains pink with eosin. Cord blood (*left*) maternal blood (*right*) with two fetal cells.

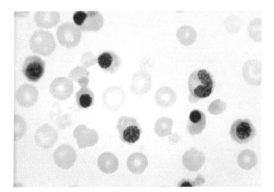

Fig. 75 HDN with nucleated red cells in the peripheral blood (*high power*).

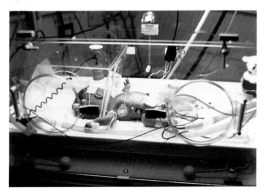

Fig. 76 Baby with HDN receiving phototherapy.

13 / Miscellaneous red cell abnormalities

Howell-Jolly bodies (Fig. 77)

These are nuclear remnants and occur predominantly following splenectomy and in hyposplenic conditions such as coeliac disease.

Following splenectomy other blood changes include the presence of target cells, occasional normoblasts and a usually transient leucocytosis and thrombocytosis.

Basophilic stippling (Fig. 78)

These are probably due to degenerate microsomes and siderosomes. They are found in lead poisoning, other toxic conditions such as severe infections and in thalassaemia.

Congenital dyserythropoietic anaemias (CDA)

This is a group of rare hereditary anaemias in which there is ineffective erythropoiesis with erythroid cell death within the marrow.

Megaloblastoid changes may occur and erythroid multinuclearity is typical. There are at least three varieties of CDA one of which (CDA II) is associated with lysis of the red cells by acidified group matched allogeneic sera (Ham's test).

Sideroblastic anaemias (Fig. 79)

These are a group of dyserythropoietic disorders in which iron-containing granules (demonstrated by Prussian blue stain) surround the nuclei of some erythroblasts. The disorder may be hereditary or acquired. The acquired form may be secondary to certain drugs (e.g. isoniazid), lead poisoning, other toxic conditions and as a clonal disorder (myelodysplasia) which may progress to acute leukaemia.

Ethanol (Fig. 80)

Excessive alcohol intake can result in dyserythropoiesis as well as morphological changes due to vitamin deficiencies.

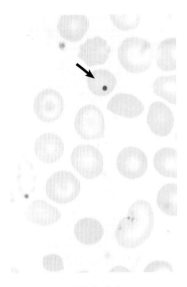

Fig. 77 Howell-Jolly body in a splenectomised patient. Note target cell to the left.

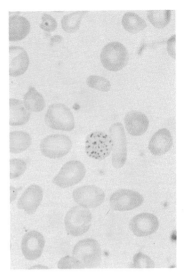

Fig. 78 Basophilic stippling.

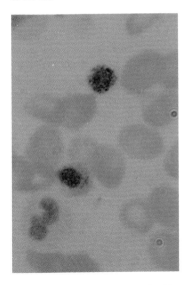

Fig. 79 Sideroblast with ringed sideroblast above (Perl's stain).

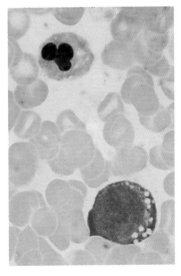

Fig. 80 Alcohol-induced dyserythropoiesis including vacuolation.

14 / Infections

Infectious mononucleosis

Aetiology This is due to infection by the Epstein-Barr herpes Virus (EBV). Young people are mainly affected. The disease is important in haematology because of the diagnostic difficulties that can arise.

Clinical features Clinically, the disease may cause non-specific malaise, fever, sore throat and lymphadenopathy (glandular fever); some cases are asymptomatic. The spleen is often palpable and there may be hepatomegaly and jaundice. Skin rashes are frequent.

A lymphocytosis develops and atypical mononuclear cells are found. These cells have irregular nuclei, often with nucleoli, but usually with condensed chromatin to distinguish them from blast cells (Figs 81 & 82). These cells are activated T cells. An autoimmune haemolytic anaemia or thrombocytopenia may also occur.

Atypical mononuclear cells are also seen in other infections including cytomegalovirus (CMV) and toxoplasmosis.

Diagnosis The diagnosis of EBV infection is dependent on the demonstration of agglutinins to horse or sheep red cells (Paul-Bunnell test; Fig. 83).

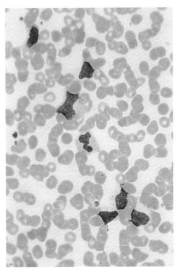

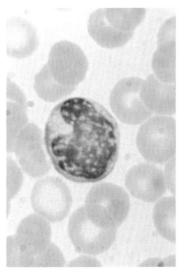

Fig. 81 Atypical mononuclear cells in infectious mononucleosis (glandular fever) with neutrophil in centre.

Fig. 82 Atypical mononuclear cell showing nuclear fenestration (*very high power*).

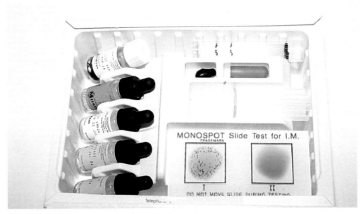

Fig. 83 Infectious mononucleosis screening test.

Human immunodeficiency virus (HIV) infection

Aetiology   Infection by the HIV virus first appears as a transient flu-like illness. There then follows a variable period of good health which may last many years. The HIV virus has tropism for cells expressing the CD4 antigen. As the disease progresses there is a steady decline in the number of CD4+ lymphocytes in the peripheral blood (Figs 84 & 85). Patients frequently develop chronic lymphadenopathy (Fig. 86) and at a later stage typically develop the signs and symptoms of chronic infections often with atypical organisms such as fungi, mycobacteria and *Pneumocystis carinii*.

Clinical features   A proportion of patients with HIV infection develop malignancies, particularly Kaposi's sarcoma, aggressive non-Hodgkin's lymphoma and Hodgkin's disease. The lymphomas frequently contain the EBV virus.

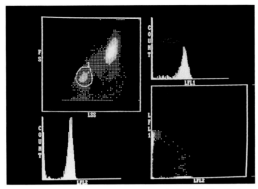

Fig. 84 Flow cytometric measurement of CD4/CD8 T-cells in a normal individual. LFL2 represents the distribution peak of CD4 stained lymphocytes and LFL1 CD8 staining. The ratio of CD4:CD8 is approximately 2:1.

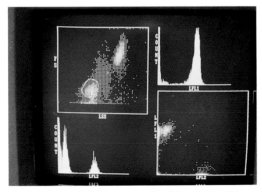

Fig. 85 Reduced CD4 cells (reverse CD4/CD8 ratio) in HIV infection.

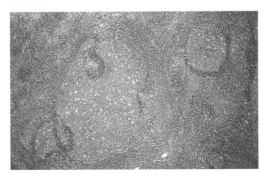

Fig. 86 Reactive lymph node in persistant glandular lymphadenopathy phase of HIV infection.

HIV infection (cont)

Patients with acquired immunodeficiency syndrome (AIDS) are often anaemic and this can be exacerbated by treatment with 5́azido-3́deoxythymidine (AZT) and cotrimoxazole (prophylaxis for pneumocystis). The neutrophil count may be reduced and in some cases this deficiency is autoimmune in origin. Immune thrombocytopenia is more common and may necessitate splenectomy.

The bone marrow in AIDS patients displays non-specific abnormalities including hypercellularity, megaloblastoid erythropoiesis (Fig. 87), myeloid dysplasia, lymphoid aggregates, eosinophilia, plasmacytosis and increased reticulin.

Diagnosis   HIV infection is diagnosed by a standard serological test, and progression can be monitored by regular measurement of CD4+ cells in the blood (Figs 84 & 85, p. 54). In the presence of fever, thorough examination and detailed investigations must be carried out to find the cause. A bone marrow examination may occasionally be the most direct way to detect mycobacterial infections or lymphoma (Figs 88 & 89).

Treatment   Therapy with AZT may slow the progress of developing AIDS, but there is as yet no highly effective specific therapy.

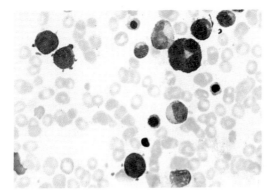

Fig. 87 Dysplastic red cell changes associated with HIV infection.

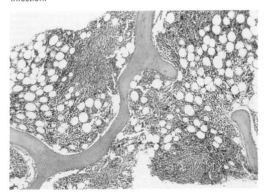

Fig. 88 Trephine section of bone marrow showing granuloma in progressive HIV infection.

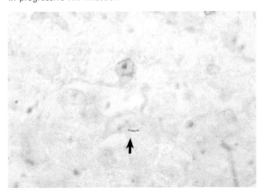

Fig. 89 Ziehl-Neelsen (ZN) stain of granuloma in HIV showing tuberculus bacillus (*arrowed*) (*high power*).

Malaria

Aetiology Malaria is due to infection with specific protozoa of the *Plasmodium* genus. It is transmitted by the bite of the *Anopheles* mosquito. The plasmodia undergo a single sexual cycle in the mosquito and recurrent asexual cycles, with the production of sexual forms (gametocytes) in man.

Clinical features The initial incubation period is 9–11 days. The disease is characterized by fever, anaemia and splenomegaly. The fever is often periodic, the frequency in part reflecting the species of *Plasmodium*. In severe cases especially of the malignant tertian form (*P. falciparum*) there may be haemolysis, thromboses, shock, cerebral intravascular coagulation.

Investigations During an acute episode there may be anaemia and plasmodial forms can be detected in the peripheral blood especially on thick films. Differentiation of the different species requires considerable expertise but is important as together with the geographical source of origin, this will influence the choice of therapy.

P. vivax (benign tertian) (Figs 91–93)
Ring forms (trophozoites) and segmented schizonts may be seen. The schizonts may develop into free merozoites or into round sexual forms (gametocytes). The invaded red cells are increased in size and contain 'Schuffner's dots'.

P. ovale (tertian) (Fig. 95, p. 60)
The appearances in the blood are similar to *P. vivax* except that the gametocytes and infected red cells are often oval with fimbriated edges. Schuffner's dots are conspicuous.

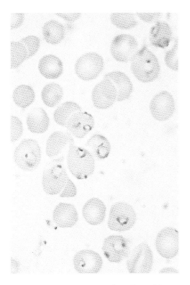

Fig. 90 Heavy malarial infestation with more than one parasite in some cells (*P. falciparum*).

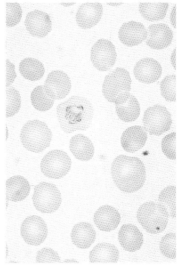

Fig. 91 *P. vivax* trophozoite. Note amoeboid form and enlargement of red cell.

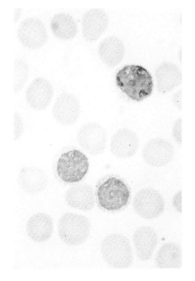

Fig. 92 Two *P. vivax* gametes and schizont (above).

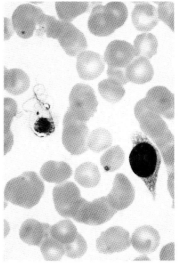

Fig. 93 Exflagellating gametocyte stage of *P. vivax* life cycle—a rare finding.

Malaria (cont)

P. malariae (quartan)

In this form the trophozoites are often band shaped. The infested red cells are not enlarged and there are no Schuffner's dots.

P. falciparum (Figs. 90, 94)

Parasites may be scanty, but red cells super-infected with trophozoites may be seen. Infected red cells are round, of normal size and Schuffner's dots are not seen. The gametocytes are typically elongated or crescentric in shape.

It should be noted that mixed infections can occur.

Treatment
Prophylaxis: This involves mosquito control, avoidance of bites and appropriate prophylactic drug therapy.

Therapy: Rest and fluids are required during the acute phase. Drugs are given to eradicate the asexual blood-borne cycle and the exoerythrocytic (liver) parasites (does not occur with *P. falciparum*). Eight groups of drugs are available and the correct drug should be chosen by an expert. Chloroquine is most commonly used.

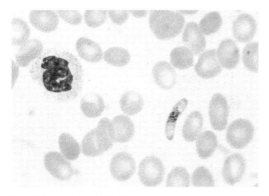

Fig. 94 Banana-shaped *P. falciparum* gamete.

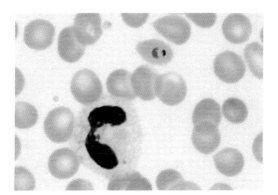

Fig. 95 Ring form *of P. ovale*. The infected erythrocyte is oval in shape with a fimbriated edge.

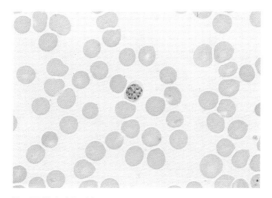

Fig. 96 Malarial schizont.

Parasites

Other parasites in the blood
Many other parasites can be detected in the blood. They include trypanosomes (Fig. 97), microfilaria (Fig. 98), and spirochaetes. *Leishmania donovani* may be found in bone marrow monocytes (Figs 99 & 100).

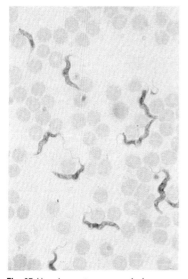

Fig. 97 Very heavy trypanosomiasis infestation.

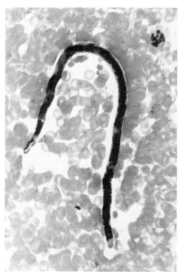

Fig. 98 Filariasis (*Loa loa*).

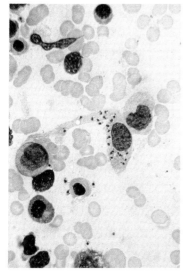

Fig. 99 *Leishmania donovani* (LD bodies) in a bone marrow macrophage.

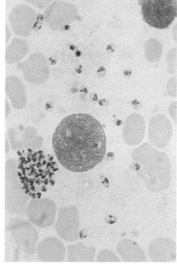

Fig. 100 *Leishmania donovani* bodies in a macrophage (splenic needle aspirate).

15 / Miscellaneous leukocyte abnormalities

Pelger-Hüet anomaly

This is an autosomal dominant condition found in 1 in 6000 individuals. Neutrophils contain not more than two lobes to the nuclei and 'band forms' are frequent (Fig. 101).

Similar morphological appearances (pseudo Pelger forms) may be seen in myeloproliferative disorders, severe infections and some other toxic conditions.

LE cells

LE cells are neutrophils that have ingested lymphocyte nucleii coated with and denatured by antibody to nucleoprotein (Fig. 102). They are produced in vitro by incubating blood at room temperature while rotating with glass beads. Lupus erythematosus (LE) cells are found in systemic lupus erythematosus (SLE) and other collagen diseases. The test has been largely replaced by the antinuclear factor test (ANF) and DNA binding assays.

Chronic granulomatous disease (CGD)

This is a rare inherited disease but is of importance as the study of the condition has helped in the understanding of the phagocyte oxidase system. The inheritance is most commonly X-linked. Affected individuals suffer from recurrent infections particularly with staphylococci. There is a poorly explained failure to switch off the inflammatory reaction with formation of granuloma in many sites and poor wound healing (Fig. 103).

Diagnosis is made by the demonstration of an inability of the neutrophils to reduce nitroblue tetrazolium dye (NBT test; Fig. 104), and the defect can be further defined by molecular techniques.

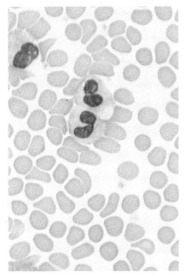

Fig. 101 Pelger-Hüet anomaly.

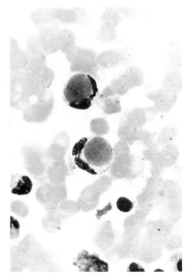

Fig. 102 LE cells.

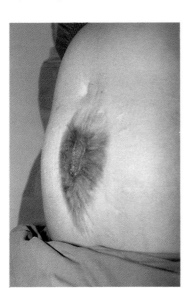

Fig. 103 Unhealed splenectomy scar in chronic granulomatous disease (CGD).

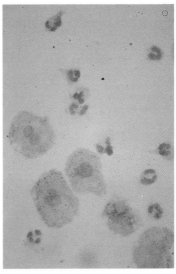

Fig. 104 Nitroblue tetrazolium test for CGD. Heterozygote pattern showing unreacting neutrophils (CGD) and neutrophils with normal redox activity (blue, swollen cells.)

Chediak–Higashi syndrome	This is a very rare autosomal recessive condition in which there is albinism, a bleeding tendency, susceptibility to bacterial infections and often progressive neurological disease. Eosinophilic inclusions are seen in the blood cells (Fig. 105).
Sea blue histiocytes	These are large lipid-containing histiocytes in the marrow which stain sea blue in colour (Fig. 106). They may be found in a rare autosomal condition characterized by neurological impairment and splenomegaly. More commonly they are found in the myeloproliferative disorders, congenital haemolytic anaemias and some chronic inflammatory disorders. The occasional sea blue histiocyte may be a normal finding.
Gaucher's disease	This is an autosomal recessive condition most common in Jews. There is β-glucocerebrosidase deficiency leading to hepatosplenomegaly, and bony infiltration. The course of the disease is very variable. The blood film often shows features of hypersplenism and typical Gaucher cells are found in the marrow (Figs 107 & 108). Specific enzyme replacement therapy is available but is very expensive.
Langerhan's cell histiocytoses	This is a group of diseases ranging from the relatively benign unifocal eosinophilic granuloma, to the multifocal variant, to the very malignant diffuse histiocytic infiltration previously known as the Letterer-Siwe syndrome. The latter condition is frequently fatal.

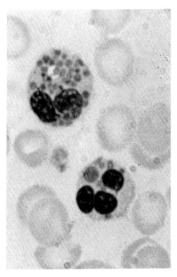

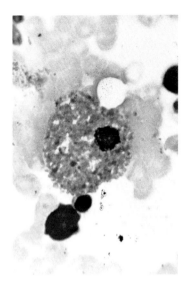

Fig. 105 Large eosinophilic granules in leukocytes in Chediak–Higashi syndrome (*very high power*).

Fig. 106 Sea blue histiocyte.

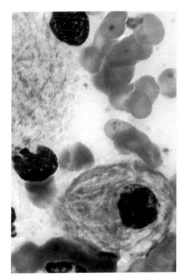

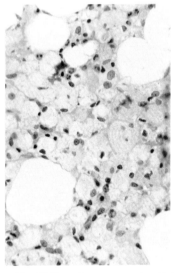

Fig. 107 Gaucher cell on marrow smear with 'onion skin' appearance.

Fig. 108 'Foamy' appearance of multiple Gaucher cells on marrow biopsy.

16 / Chronic myeloproliferative disorders

Chronic myeloid leukaemia (CML)

Aetiology

There is a malignant transformation of the multipotential haemopoietic stem cells. There are excessive cells in the granulocytic series, although initially these malignant cells do differentiate nearly normally (Fig. 109).

Clinical features of chronic phase CML

Occurs predominantly in adults. There is insidious onset of:

• Anorexia and weight loss.
• Symptoms of anaemia.
• Splenomegaly which may be massive ± spleen pain.

Investigations

• Raised WBC (Fig. 110) with immature forms in the blood and often increased eosinophils and basophils (Fig. 113, p. 70).
• The neutrophil alkaline phosphatase score is low (Fig. 112).
• The Hb is often initially normal and then falls.
• Platelet count up or down.
• Marrow hypercellular with gross myeloid hyperplasia.

Chromosomes

Philadelphia chromosome (translocation of long arm of 22 to long arm of 9) present in over 85% of cases. This results in activation of a hybrid bcr-abl proto-oncogene which can be detected by reverse transcriptase polymerase chain reaction.

Treatment in chronic phase

• Supportive, e.g. transfusions, treatment of infections, allopurinol for gout.
• Chemotherapy to normalize white blood count (WBC). Hydroxyurea or α interferon. These are not curative.
• Bone marrow transplantation from an HLA-identical sibling can be curative and should be considered in first chronic phase.

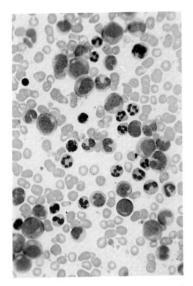

Fig. 109 Peripheral blood film (*low power*) in CML.

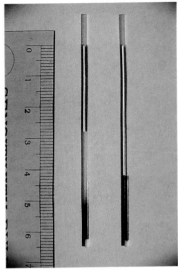

Fig. 110 Massive white cell component ('buffy coat') seen in centrifuged blood of CML (*left*) compared to normal (*right*).

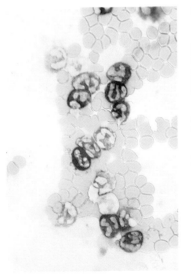

Fig. 111 NAP stain of blood film in infection (*med power*) showing neutrophil staining grades from negative (zero) to full (grade 4) intensity.

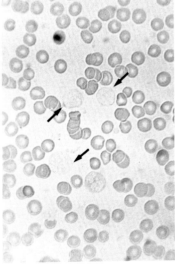

Fig. 112 NAP stain of blood film in chronic phase CML showing negative granulocytes.

Clinical features of acute phase CML

Transition to acute phase usually occurs within a few years. This may manifest as:

- increasing malaise
- increasing anaemia
- infections and fevers
- bleeding
- bone pain
- failure to respond to the usual chemotherapy.

Investigations

A fall in Hb, platelet count, a rise in the basophil count or NAP score or the development of an additional chromosome abnormality may herald transformation. In blast crisis there is a steady accumulation of blast cells. These are usually myeloblasts (Fig. 114) but lymphoid blast crisis occurs in about 20% of cases (Fig. 115). Myelofibrotic crisis occurs in some.

Treatment in acute phase CML

As for acute leukaemia. Remissions are short lived. In the early stages of transformation some cases may be salvaged by bone marrow transplantation.

Chronic myeloid leukaemia in childhood

This may resemble adult disease, but classical 'juvenile CML' is Philadelphia chromosome negative, and is characterized by a prominent monocytosis and a high HbF level.

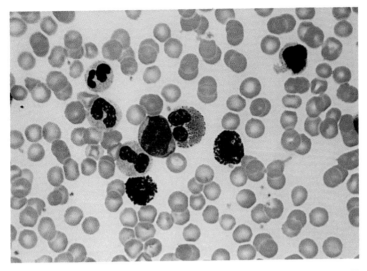

Fig. 113 Peripheral blood film (medium power) in CML showing eosinophilia, basophilia and central blast cell.

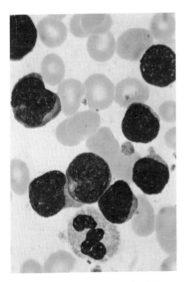

Fig. 114 Lymphoid blast crisis in CML (*high power*).

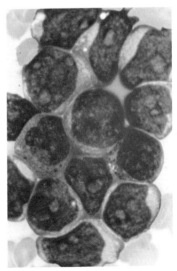

Fig. 115 Myeloid blast crisis in CML (*high power*). One blast cell showing a positive myeloperoxidase reaction.

Chronic myelomonocytic leukaemia (CMML)

This disorder is classified here as a myeloproliferative disorder but it is frequently classified as a form of myelodysplasia (pre-leukaemia).

The disorder presents insidiously with the symptoms of anaemia, fever, anorexia and weight loss. There is anaemia often with a raised MCV. Moderate leucocytosis is usually present with an increase of both granulocytic cells and monocytes, many of which may be abnormal in appearance (Figs 116 & 117). The bone marrow is hypercellular with an increase in primitive myeloid cells. The number of monocytic cells in the marrow is often surprisingly low.

This disease ultimately progresses to an acute myeloid leukaemia.

Polycythaemia rubra vera (PRV)

Aetiology There is a malignant transformation of the multipotential stem cell with excess production of red cells. There is no Philadelphia chromosome.

Clinical features Symptoms develop gradually and include:

- headaches, dizziness, tinnitus and visual problems
- thrombotic episodes
- bleeding episodes especially peptic ulcers.
- generalized pruritis
- gout.

Splenomegaly is present in 75%. One-third of patients are hypertensive.

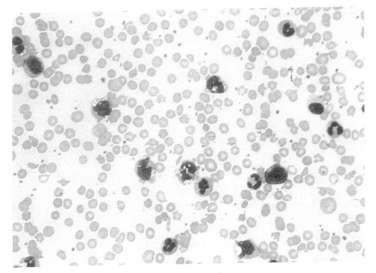

Fig. 116 Peripheral blood film in CMML (*low power*).

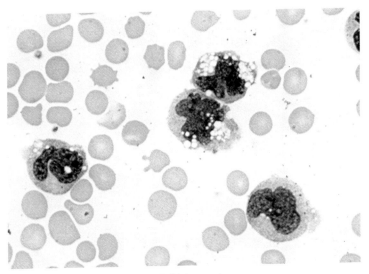

Fig. 117 Peripheral blood film in CMML (*high power*).

PRV (cont)

Investigations
- Raised Hb.
- Raised red cell mass. This is essential for the diagnosis to differentiate it from pseudopolycythaemia due to a low plasma volume.
- White count usually raised.
- NAP score raised (Fig. 118).
- Platelet count often raised.

In some cases the diagnosis of PRV must be made by careful exclusion of secondary polycythaemia. This includes a CXR, IVU, blood gases, Hb electrophoresis and O_2 dissociation curve.

Treatment
- Repeated phlebotomies.
- Chemotherapy e.g. hydroxyurea.
- Radioactive phosphorus (rarely used).
- Allopurinol to prevent gout.
- Control of blood pressure if raised.

Prognosis
Untreated PRV is fatal within several years. Treated, most patients will live for over 10 years from diagnosis. Some cases terminate in acute leukaemia or myelofibrosis.

Essential thrombocytosis

In this myeloproliferative disorder, excessive platelet production predominates (Figs 119 & 120). Patients particularly suffer from a combined bleeding and clotting tendency, as well as the general features of myeloproliferative diseases such as anaemia and malaise. Myelofibrosis is common. The diagnosis can be difficult to differentiate from reactive thrombocytosis and is partly a diagnosis of exclusion.

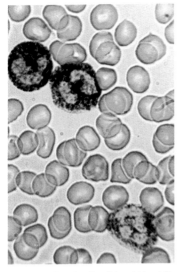

Fig. 118 NAP stain of peripheral blood film in PRV showing increased staining (*high power*).

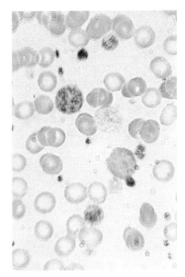

Fig. 119 Large and agranular platelet forms in essential thrombocytosis.

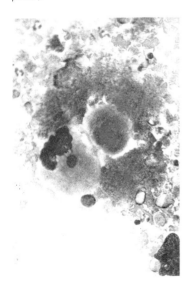

Fig. 120 Bone marrow film (*low power*) in essential thrombocythaemia showing increased megakaryocytes and drifts of platelets.

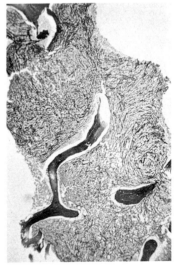

Fig. 121 Trephine biopsy stained for reticulin showing severe fibrosis.

Primary myelofibrosis

In this variety of myeloproliferative disease marrow
fibrosis (Fig. 121, p. 74, and Fig. 122) and
extramedullary haemopoiesis predominate. The
fibrosis is probably reactive. The spleen is often very
large. There is anaemia with anisocytosis and
poikilocytosis and 'tear drop' red cells. Immature red
and white cells are present in the blood
(leukoerythroblastic; Figs 123 & 124). The NAP
score is raised. Treatment is mainly supportive with
transfusion and allopurinol. Splenectomy is
occasionally indicated. Mean survival is about 5 years.
Occasionally myelofibrosis follows an acute course and
in these cases there is usually an underlying acute
megakaryoblastic leukaemia (M7).

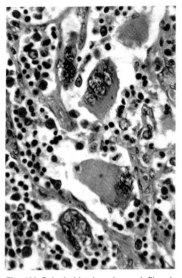

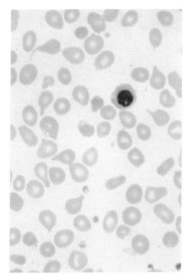

Fig. 122 Splenic histology in myelofibrosis showing extramedullary haemopoiesis. Megakaryocytes are readily seen.

Fig. 123 'Tear drop' poikilocystosis in myelofibrosis.

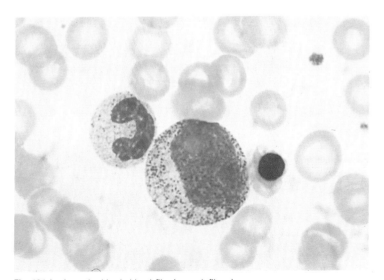

Fig. 124 Leukoerythroblastic blood film in myelofibrosis.

17 / Acute lymphoblastic leukaemia (ALL)

There is a malignant proliferation of lymphoblasts within the blood and marrow (Fig. 125). The disease is usually rapidly progressive if untreated.

Clinical features The incidence of ALL peaks in childhood and then remains relatively constant at lower levels throughout adult life.

It is slightly more common in males. It usually presents with the symptoms of sudden onset marrow failure:

- Anaemia → weakness and lethargy.
- Leucopenia → infections.
- Thrombocytopenia → purpura and bleeding.
- Bone and joint pain may occur.
- On examination, lymphadenopathy and hepatosplenemegaly are frequent.
- A mediastinal mass may be present on CXR (T-cell disease) (Fig. 126).
- CNS involvement is rare at presentation though common in late stages of the disease.

Investigations Anaemia is usual. The total leucocyte count is usually raised with lymphoblasts present. The neutrophil count is usually reduced. The platelet count is usually low. The bone marrow is hypercellular consisting almost entirely of lymphoblasts.

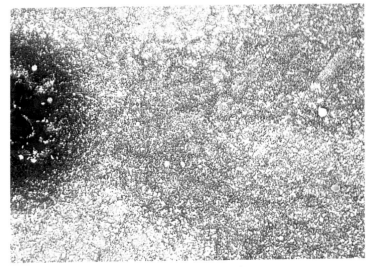

Fig. 125 Hypercellular leukaemic marrow film (*low power*).

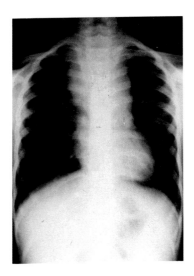

Fig. 126 Mediastinal mass in a child with T-cell ALL.

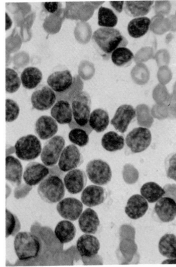

Fig. 127 ALL (*medium power*). FAB Type L_1.

Morphology and cytochemistry of lymphoblasts

Lymphoblasts generally have a very high nuclear to cytoplasmic ratio. The nuclear chromatin pattern is generally diffuse and there are one or two nucleoli which may be poorly visible.

The lymphoblasts are Sudan black and peroxidase negative (myeloid markers).

Most cases are non-specific esterase negative (granulocytic and especially monocytic marker) although T-cell ALL may shown strong polar positivity with esterase or acid phosphatase enzyme staining (Figs 128 & 129). The periodic-acid (PAS) stain is often positive (Fig. 130).

Classifications

ALL can be divided into three types on morphological criteria (French American British Classification—FAB):

L_1: Most cells are small with little cytoplasm and indistinct nucleoli. This is the most common variety (Fig. 132, p. 82).

L_2: Cells tend to be larger with relatively more cytoplasm. Nuclei often clefted with prominent nucleoli (Fig. 133, p. 82).

L_3: Large blasts with very blue cytoplasm with prominent vacuoles. These blasts are like those found in Burkitt's lymphoma (Fig. 134, p. 82). This variety is rare.

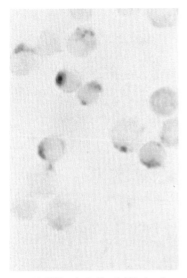

Fig. 128 NSE stain in T cell ALL showing positive polarity.

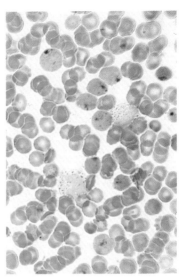

Fig. 129 Acid phosphatase stain in T cell ALL showing polar positivity.

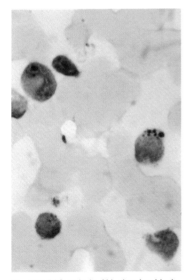

Fig. 130 PAS stain in ALL showing block positivity (*high power*).

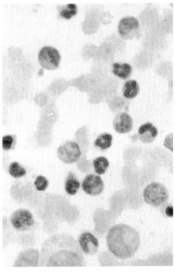

Fig. 131 PAS stain of normal marrow (*medium power*) showing diffusely positive granulocytes.

Chromosomes   Chromosome abnormalities occur in approximately one half. Hyperdiploidy is associated with a favourable prognosis. The presence of the Philadelphia chromosome t(9;22) is a poor prognostic feature and is found in 10%–30% of adult cases.

Most cases have the phenotype of immature B cells and are positive for:

- Terminal deoxynucleatidyltransferase (Tdt) (Fig. 135, p. 84)
- HLA-DR
- CD19
- Common ALL antigen (CD10) (Fig. 136, p. 84)
- About 10% of cases have an early T-cell phenotype:
  —Tdt positive
  —HLA-DR negative
  —CD10 positive or negative
  —anti-T cell antibodies positive, e.g. cytoplasmic CD3, CD7 (Fig. 135, p. 84).

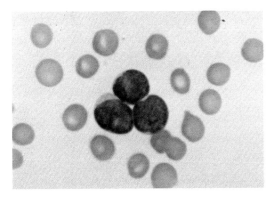

Fig. 132 ALL FAB Type L$_1$.

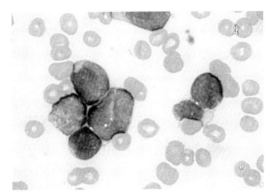

Fig. 133 ALL FAB Type L$_2$.

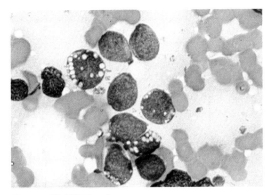

Fig. 134 ALL FAB Type L$_3$.

Treatment **Supportive:** this includes transfusion for anaemia, treatment of infections, platelets for bleeding, and social and psychological support.

Remission induction: vincristine and prednisone are used sometimes with an anthracycline (e.g. daunorubicin) in addition. Remission is obtained in over 90% of children and adults. Remission is defined as a normal blood count with less than 5% blasts in the marrow.

Maintenance / consolidation: cycles of drug therapy including vincristine, prednisone, 6-mercaptopurine and methotrexate are continued for several years after remission is obtained.

Craniospinal prophylaxis: cranial irradiation (2400 r) and intrathecal methotrexate are usually given early in remission. High dose intravenous methotrexate is an alternative form of CNS prophylaxis in low/standard risk disease. Without prophylaxis CNS disease occurs in approximately half.

Prognosis Over 65% of children with ALL are cured, in adults the cure rate is approximate 20%. Poor prognostic features include:

- high counts (>20 000) at presentation
- age <2 years or over 10 years
- males
- T-cell disease and to a lesser extent null cell disease
- L_3 variant
- presence of Philadelphia chromosome.

Bone marrow transplantation (BMT)
Once relapse has occurred, death is usual with conventional therapy. A significant proportion of these patients can be rescued with BMT from an HLA-identical sibling. BMT may also have a role in poor prognosis disease during first remission.

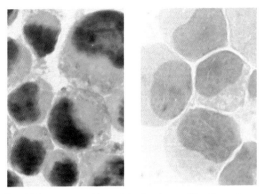

Fig. 135 Immunoperoxidase stain showing positive (brown) nuclear staining for Tdt on left but no reaction for cytoplasmic CD3 (right) in a case of B-lineage ALL.

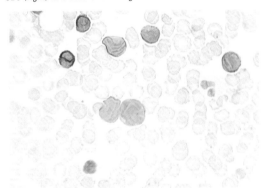

Fig. 136 Immunoperoxidase stain for the CD10 (common ALL) antigen showing positive (brown) membrane reaction.

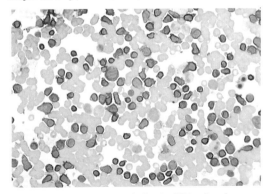

Fig. 137 Immunoperoxidase stain for the CD7 antigen in a case of T-ALL.

18 / Acute myeloblastic leukaemia (AML)

There is malignant proliferation of myeloblasts in the blood and marrow.

Clinical features

Commonest in the middle aged and elderly. Although the onset is usually acute there is a smouldering or 'preleukaemic' phase in about 15%. The presenting features of AML, as in ALL, are generally those of marrow failure:

• anaemia → weakness and lethargy
• leukopenia → infections
• thrombocytopenia → purpura and bleeding.

Bleeding may be particularly severe in acute promyelocytic leukaemia in which disseminated intravascular coagulation is a feature. Hepatosplenomegaly but not lymphadenopathy is common. Infiltration of the gums and perineum is a feature of AML.

Investigations

Anaemia is usually present. Anisocytosis and poikilocytosis are common. The white cell count is usually raised with myeloblasts the predominant cell type. Neutropenia is usual. The platelet count is usually low. The bone marrow is hypercellular and aspiration may be difficult. Blast cells predominate. Features of dyserythropoiesis and dysgranulopoiesis are seen.

In the 'preleukaemic phase' there is depression of one or more cell lines in the blood with few if any blast cells present. In the marrow there is usually marked dyshaemopoiesis and there may or may not be a modest increase in blast cells. Ringed sideroblasts may be seen on iron stains.

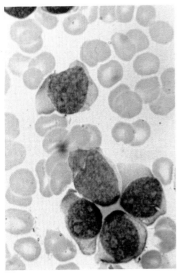

Fig. 138 Marrow film of AML (*high power*) with undifferentiated blast cells.

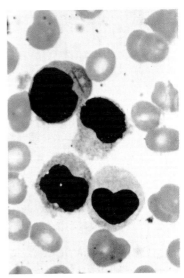

Fig. 139 AML (*high power*) with typical Auer rods.

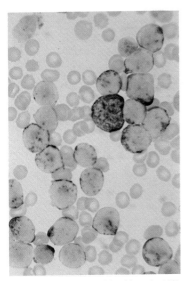

Fig. 140 Peroxidase-positive blasts in AML. The majority of blasts in this case are positive.

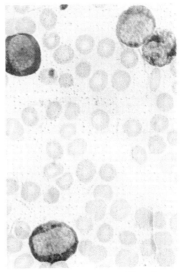

Fig. 141 Sudan black-positive blasts in AML.

Morphology and cytochemistry of myeloblasts

Myeloblasts vary in size but are usually intermediate or large cells with relatively abundant blue cytoplasm. The nuclear chromatin is finely dispersed with often more than two nucleoli per cell. The finding of 'Auer rods' (Fig. 139, p. 86) is pathognomonic of AML. Monoblasts are usually large cells with voluminous cytoplasm which may contain azurophil granules. The nucleus is often folded and contains 3–5 nucleoli.

It is difficult in some cases to differentiate myeloblasts from lymphoblasts and cytochemistry (and immunophenotype analysis) may then be helpful. Myeloblasts are typically Sudan black and peroxidase positive and PAS negative (Fig. 142) (cf. lymphoblasts) Myeloblasts are often diffusely positive for non-specific esterase (NSE) and this staining is resistant to inhibition by sodium fluoride. Monoblasts are more strongly positive for NSE (Fig. 150, p. 92) and are fluoride sensitive. Monoblasts show variable patterns of staining for peroxidase and they may be weakly PAS positive.

Classification

AML is classified according to the type of differentiation shown by the leukaemic cells (French American British—FAB classification) (Figs 138–153):

MO: Primitive blast cells showing no features of myeloid differentiation by light microscope morphology or cytochemistry. The diagnosis is based on electron microscopic cytochemistry or the expression of myeloid antigens.

M1: Blasts show few signs of maturation though a proportion are Sudan black / peroxidase positive.

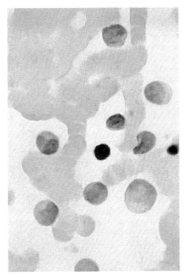

Fig. 142 PAS-negative blasts in AML. Note positive granulocyte in centre.

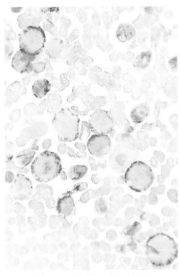

Fig. 143 Immunoalkaline phosphatase reaction showing positive (*red*) staining for the myeloid CD33 antigen.

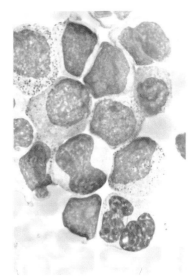

Fig. 144 AML blasts with evidence of differentiation beyond the promyelocyte stage. FAB Type M2.

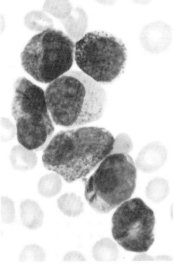

Fig. 145 Acute promyelocytic leukaemia FAB Type M3 with hypergranular promyelocytes.

Classification
(cont)

M2: Evidence of maturation at or beyond the promyelocyte stage.

M3: The majority of cells are abnormal promyelocytes with heavy granulation (acute promyelocytic leukaemia).

M4: Both granulocytic and monocytic differentiation is present, the latter being found in over 20% of cells.

M5: Pure monoblastic/monocytic differentiation.

M6: Over 30% of the nucleated cells in the marrow are erythroblasts; usually with bizarre features (acute erythroleukaemia). Myeloblasts are also seen.

M7: Megakarocyte differentiation is usually diagnosed by expression of platelet glycoproteins (e.g. CD41). Myelofibrosis is common.

Chromosomes

Abnormalities are seen in at least 50% of cases. With special techniques abnormalities may be detectable in nearly all cases; t(15; 17) and t(8; 21) are good prognostic features whereas trisomy 8 and monosomy 7 are indicative of poor prognosis disease.

Immuno-
phenotype

Myeloblasts are usually:

• Tdt negative
• HLA DR positive
• lymphoid antigen negative.
• Myeloblasts and monoblasts usually express the CD33 antigen (Fig. 143, p. 88). Erythroblasts usually stain with antiglycophorin antibodies. Monocytic-specific antibodies have also been described.

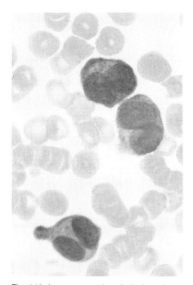

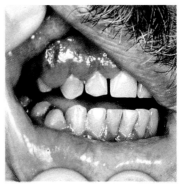

Fig. 146 Acute promyelocytic leukaemia—microgranular variant. Note 'dumbell' nuclear forms. Showing granular bundles.

Fig. 147 Gum infiltration in acute monocytic leukaemia.

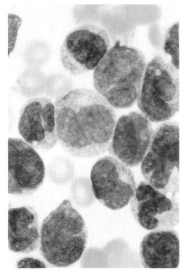

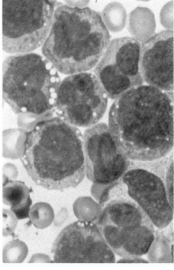

Fig. 148 Acute myelomonoblastic leukaemia FAB Type M4.

Fig. 149 Acute monoblastic leukaemia FAB Type M5.

Treatment **Supportive:** this includes transfusion for anaemia, vigorous treatment of infections, platelets for bleeding and social and psychological support. If disseminated intravascular coagulation is present (M3) large numbers of platelets and clotting factor replacement therapy are required.

Remission induction: hypoplasia is induced with repeated combinations of drugs such as daunorubicin, cytosine arabinoiside and thioguanine or etoposide.

Consolidation: it is usual to give several further courses of intensive therapy after remission is obtained (normal blood count with <5% blast cells in the marrow)

Maintenance therapy: less toxic drugs are usually given for one or two years but their value is uncertain.

Craniospinal prophylaxis: not usually given.

Bone marrow transplantation (BMT): from an HLA-matched sibling results in about 60% long-term survival (probably cured) if performed in first remission. It is therefore the treatment of choice in adults under 40 years of age with a suitable donor. High-dose therapy with autologous transplantation reduces the relapse rate but this is balanced by the increased procedure-related mortality. BMT after relapse is the only hope of cure but the results are not as good as in first remission.

Prognosis Over 70% of adult patients achieve remission but over half relapse within 2 years and the overall long-term survival is approximately 25%. Long-term results of therapy in children are better.

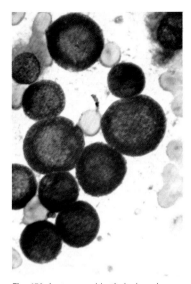

Fig. 150 Acute monoblastic leukaemia stained for non-specific esterase.

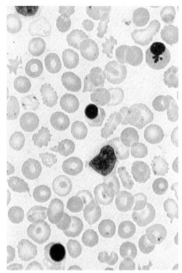

Fig. 151 Acute erythroleukaemia with bizarre red cells, normoblasts and a myeloblast in the peripheral blood. FAB Type M6.

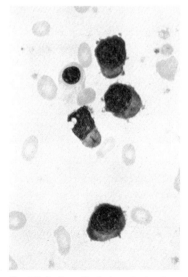

Fig. 152 Acute erythroleukaemia showing erythroblasts and myeloblasts with Auer rod.

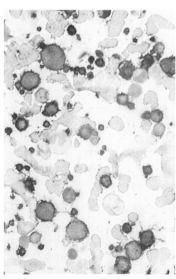

Fig. 153 Immunoalkaline phosphatase stain for platelet glycoprotein IIIa (*red reaction*) in a case of AML M7 leukaemia.

19 / Chronic lymphocytic leukaemia (CLL)

Chronic lymphocytic leukaemia is a low-grade malignancy in which there is a proliferation of small lymphocytes in the blood, marrow and lymphoid organs.

Clinical features   CLL occurs mainly in the elderly. There is usually gradual onset of fatigue, malaise and lymphadenopathy. Infections are not infrequent and bleeding problems occur in the last stages of the disease.

On examination there is usually lymphadenopathy and splenomegaly. Hepatomegaly is usually a late feature.

Investigations   There is usually a mild normocytic anaemia. This becomes more marked as the disease progresses or if there is associated autoimmune haemolytic anaemia (5–10%). The leucocyte count is usually raised with small lymphocytes predominating (Fig. 154). Most cases of CLL are B-cell neoplasms and express CD19 (Fig. 155) and CD20 but not CD10. In addition they express the CD5 antigen which is normally expressed on T cells. The cells express light-chain restricted monoclonal Ig, usually IgM ± IgD. Rare cases of CLL are T cell neoplasms. Occasional larger prolymphocytes are seen and smear cells are common. The granulocyte count and platelet count only fall late in the disease.

The bone marrow is infiltrated by small lymphocytes. Biopsy of affected lymph nodes shows a diffuse infiltration with small lymphocytes.

Hypogammaglobulinaemia occurs in one-third; 'M' bands (usually IgM) are found in approximately 5%.

A positive direct antiglobulin test occurs in 25% of cases (usually without haemolysis) at some stage during the disease.

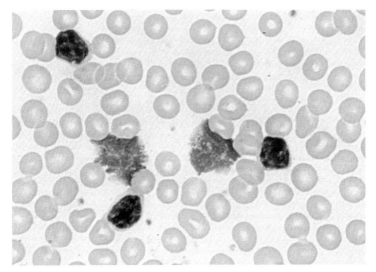

Fig. 154 Blood film of CLL (*high power*), showing smear cells.

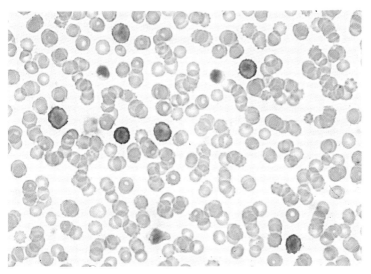

Fig. 155 Immunoalkaline phosphatase reaction for the CD19 (pan-B) cell antigen.

Treatment This disease is incurable, and asymptomatic non-progressive disease requires no therapy. When symptoms develop or the disease begins to progress, treatment with daily chlorambucil is given. Prednisone is also used especially if there is an autoimmune haemolytic anaemia. If a good response is achieved then therapy can be stopped. Ultimately resistance to chlorambucil develops and more aggressive lymphoma type therapy is required.

Prognosis The mean survival is about 5 years though some patients may survive for 10–20 years.

CLL variants

Prolymphocytic leukaemia

In this variant of CLL the malignant cells are larger than in typical CLL and the nuclei have prominent nucleoli (Fig. 156). Prolymphocytic leukaemia may be of T-cell or B-cell origin. The disease usually presents with a very high lymphocyte count, massive splenomegaly and little lymphadenopathy. This disease carries poor prognosis.

Hairy cell leukaemia

This is a low grade B-cell neoplasm in which the malignant cells have a typical hairy appearance (Fig. 157). The disease usually presents in middle age with symptoms of marrow failure and weight loss. Splenomegaly is almost invariable, hepatomegaly less common and lymphadenopathy rare.

Anaemia, neutropenia and thrombocytopenia are usual and 'hairy cells' are found in the blood. There may or may not be sufficient hairy cells to cause a lymphocytosis. A bone marrow aspirate if often difficult due to hairy cell infiltration and fibrosis. The spleen shows red cell pooling in pseudosinuses and hairy cells with a halo appearance (Fig. 158).

The disease responds well to either α interferon or deoxycoformycin. The response to standard chemotherapy is poor.

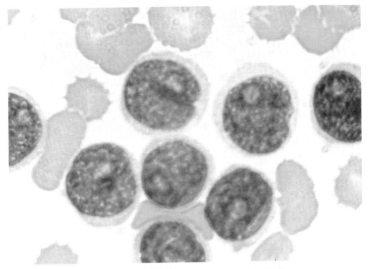

Fig. 156 Prolymphocytic variant of CLL. Showing prominant nucleoli.

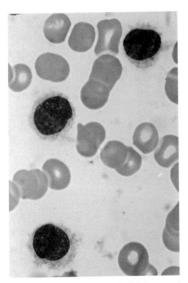

Fig. 157 Hairy cell leukaemia (*high power*).

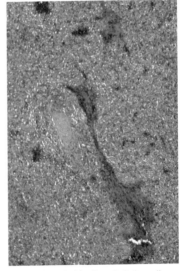

Fig. 158 Splenic histology in hairy cell leukaemia showing pseudosinuses filled with red cells.

20 / Mycosis fungoides / Sézary cell leukaemia

Mycosis fungoides (MF) and Sézary cell leukaemia (SCL) are related T-cell cutaneous lymphomas/leukaemias.

Clinical features Most common in middle-aged men. In MF there are eczematous lesions (Fig. 159) plaques (Fig. 160), tumours and ulcers of the skin without overt blood involvement. In the late stages the whole body may appear red. Lymphadenopathy is common and a leukaemic element appears (SCL); a diffuse pruritic skin rash and hepatosplenomegaly are then common. Infections frequently occur. It must be noted that some cases originate as SCL.

Investigations In SCL there is a lymphocytosis which may be over $200 \times 10^9/1$. These cells are typically large mononuclear cells with bizarre folded grooved nuclei with little cytoplasm (Figs 161 & 162). A moderate eosinophilia is common in both MF and SCL.

In SCL there is a moderate marrow infiltration with the malignant lymphocytes relative to the blood count. Skin biopsy in MF and SCL shows infiltration of the dermis by the malignant cell with the formation of so called Pautrier's microabscesses.

Treatment MF is treated with topical steroids, u/v light and psoralens, electron beam therapy or topical nitrogen mustard. Systemic therapy is given for rampant MF or SCL. Various lymphoma-type regimens are used.

Prognosis Median survival in MF is 5 years from diagnosis. The prognosis is worse in SCL.

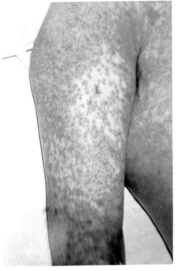

Fig. 159 Diffuse skin infiltration in Sézary's syndrome (l'homme rouge).

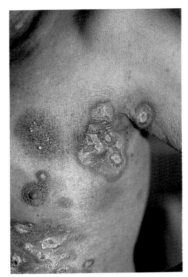

Fig. 160 Plaque of mycosis fungoides.

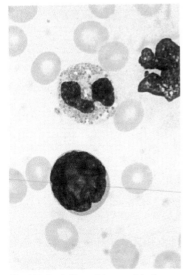

Fig. 161 Cerebriform Sézary cell in the blood.

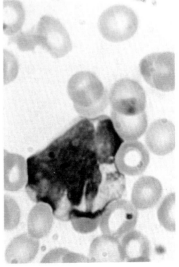

Fig. 162 Sézary cell with monstrous appearance.

21 / Multiple myeloma

This is a B-cell malignancy in which there is a proliferation of plasma cells.

Clinical features

This disease usually occurs in the elderly. The multitude of possible symptoms relate to the organ involvement in individual cases:

Marrow failure: tiredness and lethargy, infections and bleeding.

Immunoglobulin abnormalities: infections and hyperviscosity syndrome in some cases. Hyperviscosity causes lethargy, confusional states, coma, visual problems, gangrene of the extremities and a bleeding tendency.

Bone destruction: pain and hypercalcaemia in some cases. The latter can cause thirst, polyuria, constipation, abdominal pain, confusional states and coma.

Renal failure: acute or chronic renal failure. This has multiple causes including hypercalcaemia and dehydration, hyperuricaemia, amyloidosis, light chain precipitation in the tubules and urinary tract infections.

Cord compression: this is the most common abnormality. Other nerve lesions may arise due to local tumour deposits, or to amyloid. Peripheral neuropathy may also be a non-metastatic manifestation of malignancy.

Soft tissue infiltration by myeloma cells: this may cause troublesome external and internal tumours. Plasmacytomas may present without evidence of disseminated myeloma.

Investigations

Anaemia, leucopenia and thrombocytopenia are seen in varying degrees. Rouleaux are frequently seen on the film (Fig. 163), and a leucoerythroblastic picture may be present. A high ESR is usual (Fig. 164). The bone marrow shows increased plasma cells. Some appear normal and others abnormal being multinucleate or containing excessive vacuoles and inclusion bodies.

Radiographs show osteoporosis and lytic lesions in most cases (Fig. 165).

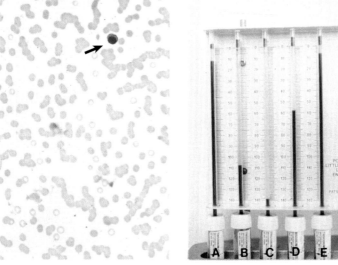

Fig. 163 Red cell rouleaux resembling pushed over piles of coins. Note plasma cell (*arrowed*) and blue background protein staining.

Fig. 164 Very high ESR in two cases of multiple myeloma (B + C). A and E are normal. D is from a patient with rheumatoid arthritis.

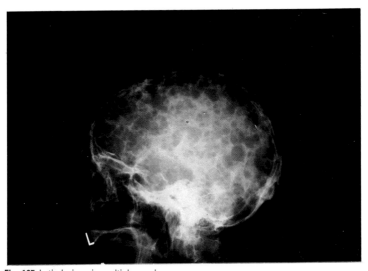

Fig. 165 Lytic lesions in multiple myeloma.

Investigations (cont)

The serum protein concentration is usually raised due to the high gammaglobulin level. The albumin level is often low. Serum protein electrophoresis usually shows a narrow monoclonal band (Fig. 166). This is usually IgG, IgA less frequently and IgD, IgE and IgM very rarely. About 20% of myelomas produce light chains only and no M band is usually detected. The immunoglobulin type can be characterized by immunoelectrophoresis. Light chains are usually present in the urine (Bence-Jones protein) and can be detected by showing that a precipitate forms at 60°C and then re-dissolves in further heating or by electrophoresis of concentrated urine.

Differential diagnosis

If lytic bone lesions, an M band and a plasmacytosis of the bone marrow (Figs 168–171) are all present then the diagnosis is not in doubt. Difficulties can arise when only one or two of these features are present.

M bands are seen in Waldenström's macroglobulinaemia, cryoglobulinaemia, CLL and some other lymphoproliferative diseases, and an M band may also be benign in which case the paraprotein level is relatively low, (benign monoclonal gammopathy) is stable over time, and other immunoglobulin levels are normal. Bony lesions and marked plasmacytosis are not seen.

A bone marrow plasmacytosis may be seen with chronic infections, inflammation and some other malignant disease. Demonstration of light chain restriction may help to differentiate a malignant from a reactive plasma cell proliferation.

Lytic lesions occur with metastases from other tumours and rarely from other causes.

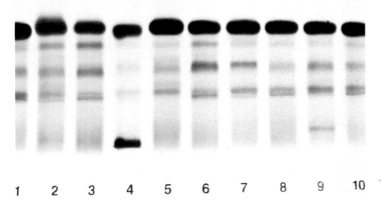

Fig. 166 Serum electrophoresis showing large (4) and small (9) M bands.

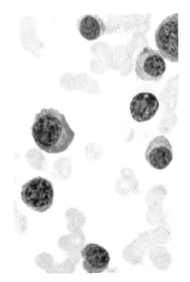

Fig. 167 Plasma cells in the bone marrow in multiple myeloma.

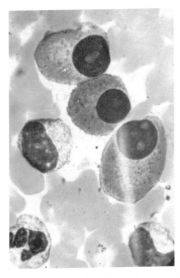

Fig. 168 Plasma cells with very basophilic/red cytoplasm in a case of IgA myeloma.

Treatment **Supportive:** fluids to correct dehydration and hypercalcaemia. The latter may also require frusemide, steroids, and sometimes mithramycin. Local radiotherapy for bone pain. Transfusion may be necessary.

Hyperviscosity responds in the short term to plasmapheresis.

Chemotherapy: myeloma is traditionally treated by melphalan but combination chemotherapy regimens may result in improved survival. A stable plateau phase (not remission) is often attained and therapy can be stopped until the disease again progresses.

Prognosis Median survival is about 2 years although some patients survive much longer.

Anaemia, uraemia, limitation of activity and a raised plasma $\beta 2$ microglobulin level are poor prognostic indicators.

Recent studies suggest that high dose therapy with autologous haematopoietic support may prolong survival although confirmation is required.

Plasmacytoma

Occasionally a solitary plasmacytoma develops, and if after a careful search there is not other evidence of dissemination, these cases can be treated by local irradiation.

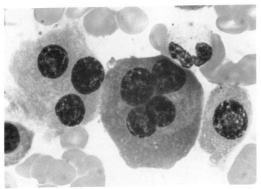

Fig. 169 Multinucleate plasma cells in myeloma.

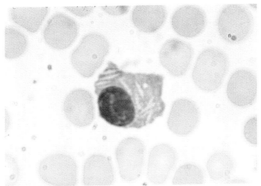

Fig. 170 Paraprotein crystals in a plasma cell.

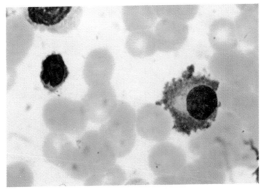

Fig. 171 'Flame' cell form of plasma cell.

22 / Waldenström's macroglobulinaemia

This is a B-cell malignancy in which there is a proliferation of small lymphocytes with some plasmacytoid differentiation (Fig. 172). There is usually massive production of monoclonal IgM.

Clinical features This is a disease of the elderly. It usually presents with symptoms of hyperviscosity. Weight loss is also common. There may be hepatosplenomegaly or lymphadenopathy (cf. myeloma). Bony lesions are not usually seen.

Investigations Anaemia and a high ESR are usual. The leucocyte count and platelet count are often normal, though malignant lymphoid cells may be seen. The bone marrow shows diffuse infiltration by plasmacytoid lymphocytes.

The serum IgM is usually very high and other immunoglobulins may be low.

Cryoglobulins and Bence-Jones proteins may be present. Plasma viscosity is usually very high. Renal impairment is unusual (cf. myeloma)

Treatment No treatment is required in cases that are relatively quiescent without symptoms. Chlorambucil or cyclophosphamide are usually given with or without steroids when chemotherapy is required. Plasmapheresis may be useful for hyperviscosity.

Prognosis Median survival is approximately 5 years.

Cryoglobulinaemia

Cryoglobulins are immunoglobulins which precipitate when cooled (Figs 173 & 174). They can give rise to Raynaud's phenomena, vascular purpura, joint pains and occasionally renal failure. The cryoglobulin may be monoclonal which is usually due to a lymphoproliferative disorder or polyclonal which is usually reactive. A mixed monoclonal and polyclonal pattern is seen in autoimmune disease. Treatment is by avoidance of cold and therapy of the underlying condition.

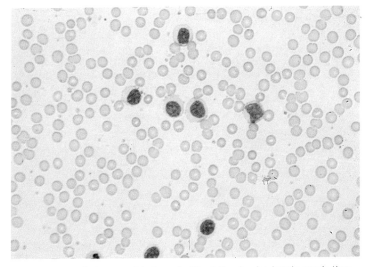

Fig. 172 Waldenström's macroglobulinaemia. Blood film showing lymphocytosis (*low power*).

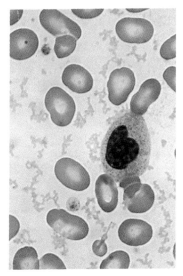

Fig. 173 Cryoglobulinaemia on blood film.

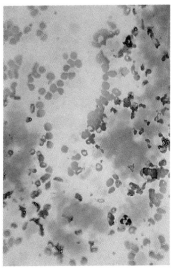

Fig. 174 Extensive cryoglobulinaemia precipitates on blood film (*low power*).

23 / Hodgkin's disease

Hodgkin's disease (HD) is a malignant neoplasm that usually arises in a lymph node. The nature of the malignant cell (Reed-Sternberg cell: RS) remains uncertain. Clonally integrated Epstein Barr virus is present in the RS cells in about 40% of cases.

Clinical features

The peak incidence of HD is in young adults.

Lymphadenopathy, especially in the neck, is the most common presenting feature. The glands may or may not be tender. Fever, night sweats, malaise, weight loss and pruritis may all occur early in the disease. Because HD can occur almost anywhere, the possible symptom complex is enormous (Fig. 175).

Investigations

Anaemia may be present, and is usually a non-specific feature of advanced disease rather than marrow infiltration. The neutrophil count and eosinophil count may be raised, or reduced if there is marked hypersplenism. The platelet count it usually normal in the early stages of cases. The serum albumin is often reduced and the serum lactate dehydrogenase (LDH) level raised in advanced diseases.

Lymph node histology (Figs 176–182)

The diagnosis is usually dependent on the histology of an affected node. The detection of RS cells and their mononuclear counterparts are of prime importance although these cells are usually a minor population surrounded by reactive lymphocytes, neutrophils, eosinophils, plasma cells, histiocytes and fibroblasts.

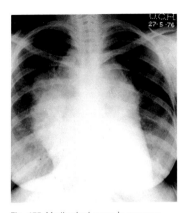

Fig. 175 Mediastinal mass in a young woman with HD.

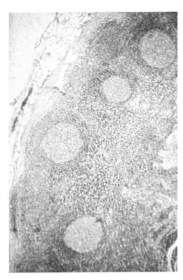

Fig. 176 Normal lymph node histology (*very low power*).

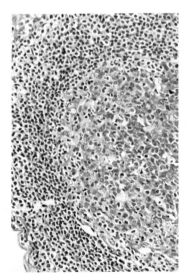

Fig. 177 Normal germinal centre (*low power*).

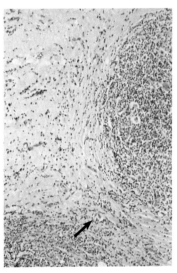

Fig. 178 Nodular sclerosing HD (*low power*) showing bands of fibrosis (*arrowed*).

RS cells are classically large binucleate cells with prominent nucleoli. They often appear to have a clear space around them. The classification of HD is largely dependent on the reactive elements in the node.

Nodular sclerosis: RS cells are readily seen and are often in lacunae. The node is divided by bands of fibrotic tissue. This is the most common variety accounting for 70%–80% of cases.

Lymphocyte predominant: RS cells are less prominent and there are large numbers of reactive lymphocytes.

Lymphocyte depleted: RS-like cells are prominent and there are few reactive lymphocytes. This entity is now rarely diagnosed and such cases are usually classified as non-Hodgkin's lymphomas.

Mixed cellularity: RS cells are readily seen and there are reactive lymphocytes, neutrophils, eosinophils and plasma cells.

Immunocytochemistry: In nodular sclerosing and mixed cellularity Hodgkin's disease the RS cells and their mononuclear counterparts do not usually express the common leukocyte antigen (CD45-) or typical B cell antigens (CD19-, CD20-, CD22-). They express CD15 and CD30. In lymphocyte predominant Hodgkin's disease, by contrast, the CD45 and B cell antigens are expressed, CD15 is negative and CD30 is negative.

Staging The Ann Arbor staging system is used:

Stage 1: Single lymph node region affected.

Stage 2: Two or more node regions affected on the same side of the diaphragm.

Stage 3: Nodes ± spleen affected on both sides of the diaphragm.

Stage 4: Involvement of the viscera or bone marrow.

Each stage is further divided into an A category without systemic symptoms and a B category with systemic symptoms. Staging requires thorough examination and investigation including CXRs and whole body CT scans. Lymphangiograms are infrequently used but can be informative. Staging laparotomy is now rarely carried out.

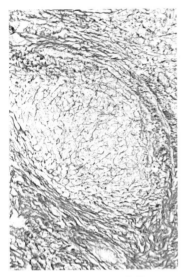

Fig. 179 Nodular sclerosing HD (*low power*), reticulin stain.

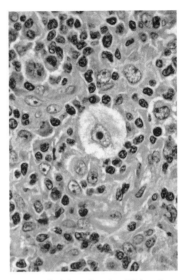

Fig. 180 Nodular sclerosing HD (*medium power*) showing lacunar cell.

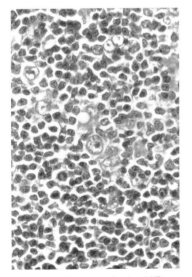

Fig. 181 Lymphocyte-predominant HD. Occasional large RS cells can be seen.

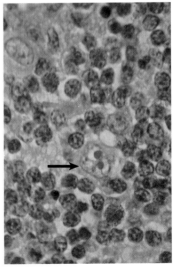

Fig. 182 Mixed cellularity HD. Note lymphocyte and eosinophil reaction and classical RS cell (*arrowed*) with 'owls eye' nucleoli.

Treatment **Radiotherapy** (3500–4000 rads) is given for most patients with stage IA or IIA disease. A mantle field is usually given for disease above the diaphragm and an inverted Y for disease below the diaphragm (Fig. 184). Local radiotherapy may be used as an alternative. This results in a higher relapse rate, but not a difference in survival.

Chemotherapy is given for all stages except IA and IIA, and is also given to those relapsing after radiotherapy. Alternating cycles of theoretically non-cross resistant agents are usually given (e.g. MOPP alternating with ABVD). Therapy is continued for about 6 months. For selected patients failing standard chemotherapy, high-dose chemotherapy with autologous haemopoietic stem cell support probably affords the best chance of long-term survival.

Prognosis Stages I and II have a good prognosis compared to III and IV. B symptoms, anaemia, a high ESR, a low lymphocyte count, low albumin and a raised LDH level are poor prognostic features. Overall a complete remission is obtained in about 80% and approximately 60% are alive and well at 10 years.

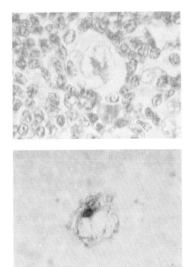

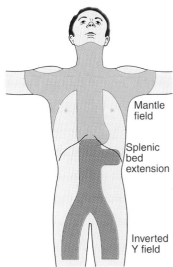

Fig. 183 CD15 immunoperoxidase stain.

Fig. 184 Radiotherapy fields for the treatment of HD.

Mantle field

Splenic bed extension

Inverted Y field

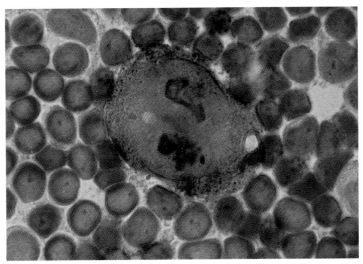

Fig. 185 CD30 + (Ki −1) Hodgkin's cell.

24 / Non-Hodgkin's lymphomas

Most non-Hodgkin's lymphomas (NHL) are B-cell neoplasms though occasionally they are of T-cell lineage.

Clinical features NHL occurs mainly in the elderly, although some cases occur in childhood. Most patients have widespread lymphadenopathy at presentation (cf: HD). Hepatosplenomegaly is common. Patients with less aggressive disease often have no symptoms, whereas those with aggressive disease tend to suffer from malaise, fevers and weight loss.

Investigations Anaemia is not infrequent. Autoimmune haemolytic anaemia may occur especially in low-grade lymphomas. Neutropenia and thrombocytopenia occur if there is marrow failure, hypersplenism or an immune destruction. Malignant cells are not usually detectable in the blood although a leukaemic element may develop in the later stages. A bone marrow biopsy shows infiltration with malignant lymphoid cells in approximately 20% cases. The infiltration is usually diffuse even in 'nodular' disease, and often has a paratrabecular distribution.

Hypoalbuminaemia and hypergammaglobinaemia and M bands are not infrequent, though the M band level is usually small or moderate.

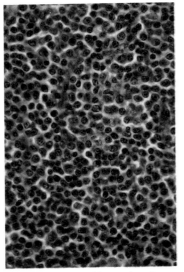

Fig. 186 Lymph node biopsy of small lymphocytic lymphoma (CLL like) (*low power*).

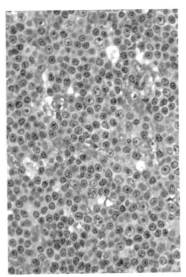

Fig. 187 Small lymphocytic lymphoma with plasmacytoid differentiation (Waldenström's like) (*low power*).

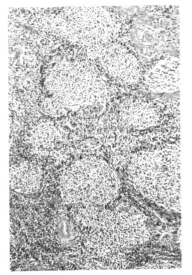

Fig. 188 Follicular lymphoma (*very low power*).

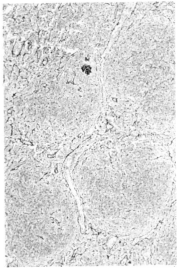

Fig. 189 Follicular lymphoma: reticulin stain.

Lymph node histology (Figs 186–196)

Many histological classifications are available illustrating their difficulty and deficiencies. The classification used below (working formulation) is based on whether or not the tumour is nodular or follicular, whether the cells are small or large and whether or not the nuclei are regular, cleaved or convoluted. Reactive elements are in general less pronounced than in HD.

Classification

Low grade
- Small lymphocytic (similar to CLL).
- Follicular predominantly small cleaved cells.
- Follicular mixed small cleaved and large cells.

Intermediate grade
- Follicular predominantly large cells.
- Diffuse small cleaved cell.
- Diffuse mixed small cleaved and large cells.
- Diffuse large cell.

High grade
- Diffuse large cell—immunoblastic.
- Lymphoblastic.
- Small non-cleaved cells (cells larger than CLL cells).

This classification does not take immunophenotype into account, although such studies do add additional information. One of the other weaknesses of this classification is that it does not take account of biological entities such as tumours of mucosa-associated lymphoid tissue (MALT).

Precise classification requires considerable expertise and experience. The most important aspect is to determine whether the disease is of low grade or intermediate/high grade and whether in the latter group there is a high risk of spread to the CNS (mainly lymphoblastic and small non-cleaved cell lymphomas) as this modifies treatment.

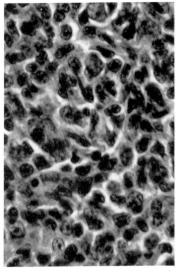

Fig. 190 Follicular lymphoma (*high power*) with a predominance of small cleaved cells.

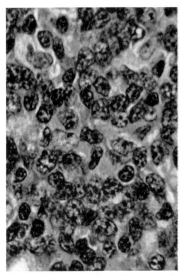

Fig. 191 Follicular lymphoma (*high power*) with a mixture of small cleaved and large cells.

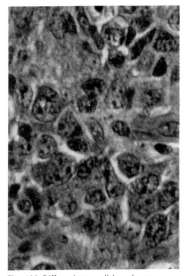

Fig. 192 Diffuse large cell lymphoma.

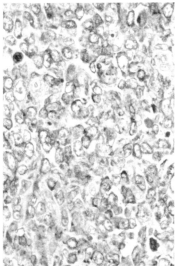

Fig. 193 Large cell lymphoma of B cell origin as shown by immunoperoxidase staining for anti-κ light chains.

Cell markers   As well as routine histological stains it is possible to perform cytochemistry and immunoperoxidase studies on paraffin embedded tissue sections. Some monoclonal antibodies will only react on frozen sections however. All follicular lymphomas are of B-cell origin as are the majority of the diffuse NHL. T-cell NHL accounts for 10–15% of the diffuse NHL. The term histiocytic lymphoma used in the Rappaport classification to refer to large cell lymphomas is misleading as lymphomas of the macrophage/histiocytic lineage are exceedingly rare.

Cytogenetics/ molecular analysis   Most follicular lymphomas have a t(14;18) translocation which results in high level expression of the bcl-2 gene with protection of such cells from apoptosis. Rearrangements of the bcl-6 gene are common in large cell lymphomas, and (t8;14) translocations are frequent in small non-cleaved cell lymphomas resulting in high level expression of the proto-oncogene c-myc.

Staging   The same staging system is used as in HD.

Treatment   Low-grade lymphomas although incurable at present, often progress very slowly, and treatment should only be given to relieve symptoms, or in a clinical trial. In the intermediate and high-grade lymphomas patients are nearly all symptomatic and more aggressive therapy is justified as there is a chance of cure.

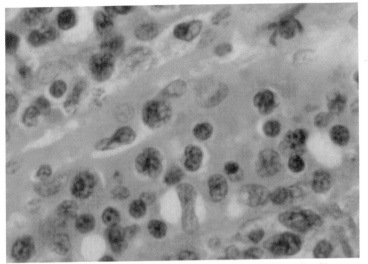

Fig. 194 T-cell lymphoblastic lymphoma invading a blood vessel. Note cells with convoluted nuclei.

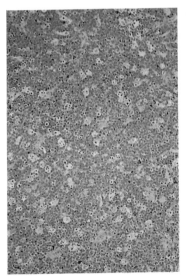

Fig. 195 Small non-cleaved cell lymphoma (*very low power*). The 'starry sky' appearance is typical of Burkitt's lymphoma.

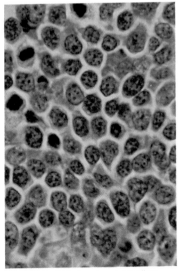

Fig. 196 Burkitt's lymphoma (*medium power*) showing small round cells with prominent nucleoli.

Treatment
(cont)

Radiotherapy (Fig. 184, p. 112): This is used mainly to reduce local node masses. Local radiotherapy may alone be curative in truly localized Stage 1 lymphomas.

Chemotherapy: In low-grade cases single agent therapy with chlorambucil or cyclophosphamide are usually used. Fludarabine may also be useful. In resistant cases more aggressive combination chemotherapy regimes can be used. In intermediate and high-grade lymphomas the trend is towards increasingly aggressive combination chemotherapy regimes. Most regimes contain cyclophosphamide, adriamycin, vincristine and prednisone (CHOP) and in some protocols bleomycin, methotrexate and cytosine arabinoside are added. Lymphoblastic lymphomas and small non-cleaved cell lymphomas require cranial prophylaxis and are therefore frequently treated on ALL type protocols.

In NHL therapy is given until complete remission, continued for several courses (consolidation) and then stopped (no maintenance).

Prognosis

Low-grade disease cannot be cured but the median survival is about 7 years. In intermediate and high-grade diseases aggressive therapy produces remissions in about 60% of patients and about half of these patients are cured.

Advanced age, Stage III and IV, poor performance status and a raised LDH all predict for a poorer outcome.

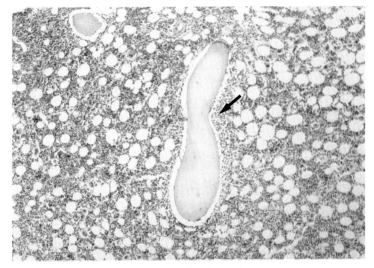

Fig. 197 Subtle paratrabecular lymphoma infiltration of the bone marrow.

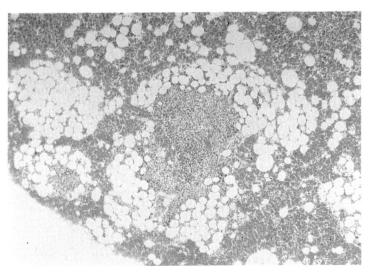

Fig. 198 Nodular infiltration of the bone marrow in follicular lymphoma.

25 / Malignant infiltration of the marrow

Many cancers may infiltrate the marrow; most common are carcinoma of the lung, breast, prostate, colon and thyroid.

The blood count may be normal although pancytopenia may occur and there may be a leukoerythroblastic blood picture.

Marrow aspirates may be difficult because of fibrosis and trephine biopsies should also be performed. The features of cancer cells (Figs 199 & 200) include:

- A tendency to form clumps.
- High nuclear to cytoplasmic ratio.
- Nuclear moulding.
- Large prominent nucleoli.

Histology Some tumours can be clearly identified by cytochemistry. Adenocarcinoma cells, for instance may stain with mucin stains.

Other tumours can be very difficult to differentiate from haematological malignancies and cell marker studies may then be useful. The CD45 antigen is expressed on most haematological tumours but not other cancers (Figs 201 & 202).

Osteosclerosis

Osteosclerosis of the bone may rarely occur as an inherited disorder (Albers-Schoenberg disease). It leads to frequent fractures, cranial nerve palsies and a leukoerythroblastic anaemia. It can be successfully treated in infancy by bone marrow transplantation. Bone sclerosis also occurs in association with primary and secondary myelofibrosis and in Paget's disease.

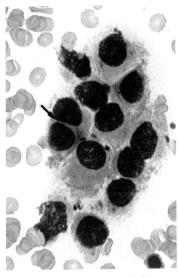

Fig. 199 Clump of malignant cells in marrow aspirate (*high power*). Some nuclear moulding apparent.

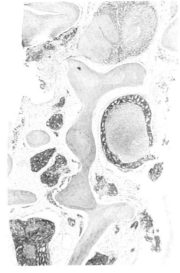

Fig. 200 Trephine biopsy showing large clumps of adenocarcinoma.

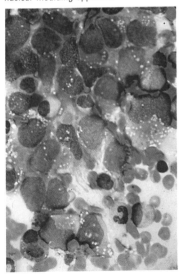

Fig. 201 May Grunwald Giemsa stain of malignant cells in bone marrow aspirate.

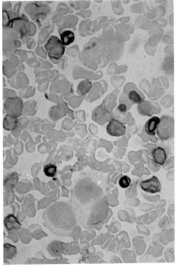

Fig. 202 Immunoperoxidase stain for the leucocyte common antigen (CD45RA) in case shown in Fig. 201. The infiltrating cells are negative and were shown subsequently to be metastatic melanoma (S100 antigen positive).

26 / Bone marrow and peripheral blood stem cell transplantation

Principle Most chemotherapy drugs used in haematological malignancies are myelosuppressive and this limits the doses of therapy that can be given. This problem can however be overcome by transplantation of haemopoietic stem cells. The stem cells may be the patient's own taken before the high-dose therapy (autologous), from an identical sibling (syngeneic) or from another individual (allogeneic). Most allogeneic donors are HLA-matched siblings but panels of HLA-typed volunteer donors are now available.

Haemopoietic stem cells were traditionally collected from the bone marrow but are now frequently obtained by leucapheresis after administration of chemotherapy and haemopoietic growth factors (e.g. G-CSF) to mobilize the stem cells into the blood (Figs 203 & 204). The stem cells can be purified on the basis of their expression of the CD34 antigen (Fig. 205). Allogeneic transplants have greater toxicity and procedure-related mortality than autografts which limits their use to younger patients (usually <45 years old). Autografts may however be contaminated by malignant cells and in the allogeneic transplant setting a significant graft vs leukaemia effect may occur.

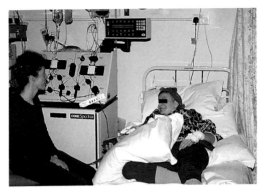

Fig. 203 Peripheral blood stem cells being collected by continuous flow apheresis following stem cell mobilization.

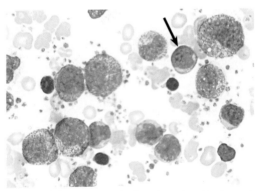

Fig. 204 MGG appearance of apheresis product showing early white cells including a blast cell (*arrowed*).

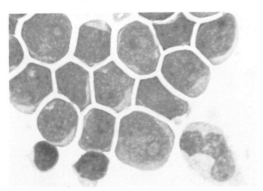

Fig. 205 Blastic appearance of purified CD34+ cells from an apheresis collection with monocyte (*bottom right*).

Indications

The indications for stem-cell transplantation are fluid as the results of conventional therapy are improving in some situations. In general allogeneic transplantation is recommended for patients with CML in first chronic phase, and in poor-risk cases of acute leukaemia in first remission, or in patients in second remission. Autologous transplantation is probably the treatment of choice for patients with HD and NHL failing standard chemotherapy. High-dose therapy and peripheral blood stem cell transplantation (PBSCT) is also being explored in solid tumours especially breast cancer.

Complications of stem cell transplantation

- Immediate period of pancytopenia lasting for 10–20 days during which bacterial and fungal infections may arise.
- Protracted immunosuppression agents. *Pneumocystis carinii* (Fig. 206) and cytomegalovirus infections are not infrequent in the first few months after transplantation. Reactivation of herpes zoster may occur in the first year following transplantation and can be disseminated (Fig. 207).
- Ablative chemo/radiotherapy is the commonest cause of veno-occlusive disease in developed countries.
- Graft versus host disease (GVHD) may cause skin (Fig. 208), gut and hepatocellular damage in the early regenerative period. In the chronic stage it gives rise to scleroderma-like changes of the skin and gut and obstructive jaundice. Acute GVHD can be minimized by T-cell depletion of the graft and cyclosporin A treatment. It may respond to steroid therapy.

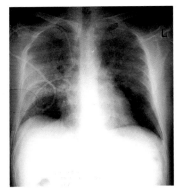

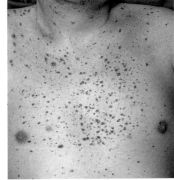

Fig. 206 Interstitial shadowing in a case of *Pneumocystis carinii*.

Fig. 207 Disseminated herpes zoster.

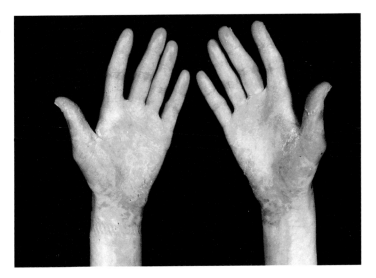

Fig. 208 Chronic graft versus host disease skin reaction.

27 / **Thrombocytopenia**

Clinical features Thrombocytopenia leads to bruising and petechial haemorrhages affecting primarily the skin and mucous membranes (Figs 209–212). Bleeding does not usually occur until the platelet count is less than $40 \times 10^9/1$.

Aetiology Thrombocytopenia may be caused by:

1. *Spurious thrombocytopenia due to platelet clumping* (Figs 213 & 214, p. 130).

2. *Decreased platelet production*
- A variety of congenital disorders including Fanconi's syndrome.
- Acquired generalized marrow hypoplasia (including cytotoxic drug therapy) or marrow infiltration.
- Viral infections.
- Drug reactions.
- Megaloblastic anaemia.

3. *Increased platelet destruction*
- Immune-mediated thrombocytopenia. This category includes some drug-induced thrombocytopenias, and idiopathic thrombocytopenia (ITP).
- Microangiopathic destruction including disseminated intravascular coagulation (DIC) and the haemolytic uraemic syndrome (HUS).
- Some infections.
- Hypersplenism.
- Following massive haemorrhage.

The two forms of true thrombocytopenia are differentiated by the number of megakaryocytes in the bone marrow.

Idiopathic thrombocytopenic purpura (ITP)

Aetiology ITP is almost invariably immune mediated. Many childhood cases follow viral infections.

Clinical features ITP tends to occur in young children as an acute self-limiting disease. In adults the disease has a more chronic course. Petechiae and bruising occur. Splenomegaly occurs rarely and its presence suggests another underlying disease.

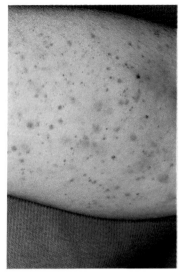

Fig. 209 Thrombocytopenic purpura.

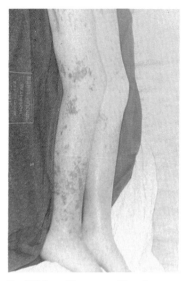

Fig. 210 Vasculitic purpura (Henoch-Schönlein purpura) resembling thrombocytopenic purpura.

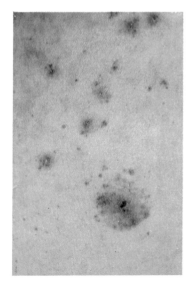

Fig. 211 Vasculitic purpura (*high power*).

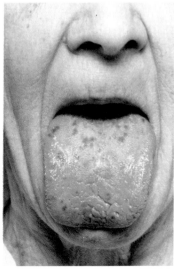

Fig. 212 Hereditary telangiectasia affecting the tongue—not purpura.

ITP (cont)

Investigations Anti-platelet antibodies can be demonstrated in most cases but the diagnosis of ITP is usually based on the history, the finding of decreased platelets without other abnormalities and increased megakaryocytes in the marrow (Fig. 215).

Treatment No treatment is required in most childhood cases although steroids are often given. In adults high-dose steroids are usually required and these can be tailed off as the response occurs. In refractory patients splenectomy is often helpful. In those patients who still do not respond, azathioprine or other immunosuppressive agents may be tried.

Disseminated intravascular coagulation (DIC)

There is widespread deposition of fibrin in the blood vessels in association with consumption of platelets and clotting factors.

Aetiology • Septicaemia.
• Shock of all types.
• Obstetric disasters.
• Promyelocytic leukaemia and other malignancies.

Clinical features This varies between a mild bleeding tendency and catastrophic oozing from all orifices and venepuncture sites.

Investigations The platelet count is reduced. There may be red cell fragmentation (Fig. 216). The thrombin time, prothrombin time and partial thromboplastin time are all prolonged. Plasma fibrinogen is reduced. Fibrin degradation products are found in blood and urine.

Treatment Treatment is primarily that of the underlying disorder with replacement of clotting factors and platelets as necessary.

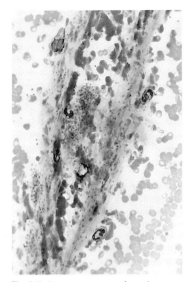

Fig. 213 A common cause of spurious thrombocytopenia—small fibrin/platelet clots on film.

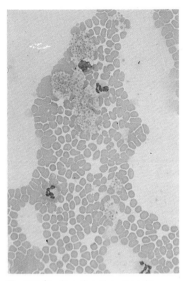

Fig. 214 Spurious thrombocytopenia; platelet clumps.

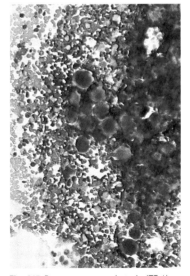

Fig. 215 Bone marrow aspirate in ITP (*low power*) showing masses of megakaryocytes.

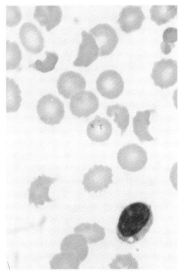

Fig. 216 Blood film in DIC showing thrombocytopenia and fragmented red cells.

28 / **Thrombocytosis**

Clinical features Thrombocytosis is usually asymptomatic but may cause thromboses. Bleeding tendencies are common in the myeloproliferative disorders with elevated platelet counts (Fig. 217).

Aetiology
- Myeloproliferative disorders, particularly essential thrombocytopenia.
- Response to blood loss or haemolysis.
- Response to stress such as surgery, especially splenectomy.
- Response to some infections and chronic inflammatory disorders, including the collagen vascular diseases.
- In association with some tumours.

The platelet count is often above $1000 \times 10^9/1$ in primary thrombocytosis but is not usually this high in the secondary varieties.

Treatment This is basically that of the underlying disease. Aspirin may help prevent digital gangrene (Fig. 218) which can occur with very high platelet counts.

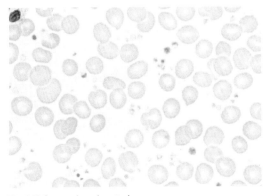

Fig. 217 Severe thrombocytosis.

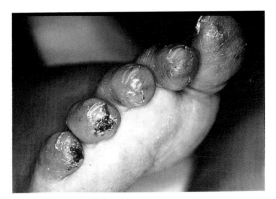

Fig. 218 Gangrene of the extremities in a case of thrombocytosis.

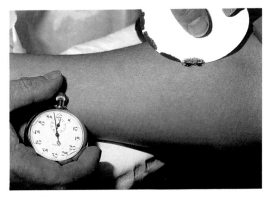

Fig. 219 Template bleeding time measurement.

Qualitative platelet defects

There are a large number of rare congenital diseases
in which the platelets function abnormally leading to
a bleeding tendency and prolonged bleeding times
(Fig. 219, p. 132). In the Bernard-Soulier syndrome
(autosomal recessive) the platelets are often very large
(Fig. 220). In the grey platelet syndrome the platelets
lack granules (Fig. 222) and myelofibrosis may occur.
In the May-Hegglin anomaly (autosomal dominant)
the platelets are normal or reduced in number, have a
large size and inclusion bodies are present in the
leucocytes (Fig. 223).

Functional platelets abnormalities may also be
acquired in association with renal failure, liver failure,
paraproteins and in the myeloproliferative disorders.
Many drugs especially aspirin, also interfere with
platelet function.

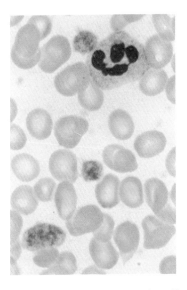

Fig. 220 Large platelets from a patient with the rare Bernard-Soulier syndrome.

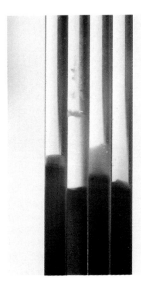

Fig. 221 Contributing factors to increased blood viscosity: normal centrifuged blood (*far right*) compared to (*from left*) increased myeloid buffy coat, paraprotein and massive platelet count.

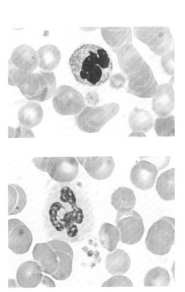

Fig. 222 Agranular platelets in a case of grey platelet syndrome compared to normal, granular platelets (*below*).

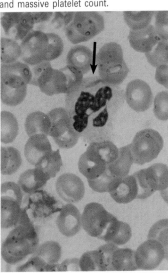

Fig. 223 May-Hegglin's anomaly—large platelets and Dohle bodies (arrowed) in the neutrophils.

29 / **Coagulation abnormalities**

Clinical features   Abnormalities in the clotting cascade lead mainly to excessive bleeding after surgery, easy bruising and bleeding into the soft tissue and joints (Figs 224–228).

Aetiology   **Congenital clotting factor deficiency**
- Factor VIII deficiency (haemophilia A).
- Von Willebrand's disease.
- Other factor deficiencies.

Acquired coagulation disorders
- Liver disease causes lack of production of the vitamin K dependent clotting factors, factor V and fibrinogen.
- Vitamin K deficiency occurs in the new-born, with malabsorption and with oral anticoagulants.
- DIC.
- Nephrotic syndrome with renal loss of some factors.
- Clotting factor inhibitors which are usually associated with administration of factor VIII, but may arise spontaneously especially in association with tumours or collagen vascular diseases.
- Heparin therapy.

Haemophilia A

Aetiology   This is an X-linked recessive disorder; it occurs in males but is carried by females. There is a severe deficiency of that part of the factor VIII molecule with clotting activity (factor VIII C).

Investigations   The partial thromboplastin time (PTT) is prolonged (intrinsic system). The prothrombin time (extrinsic system) and the thrombin time (common pathway) are normal. The defect in the PTT can be corrected by mixing with normal plasma. The diagnosis is confirmed with a specific factor VIII assay: level >5% mild disease; 1–5% moderate disease; <1% severe disease.

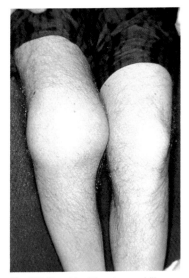

Fig. 224 Knee bleed in a haemophiliac.

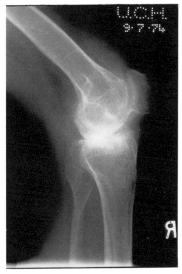

Fig. 225 Radiograph of haemophiliac knee showing severe degenerative changes.

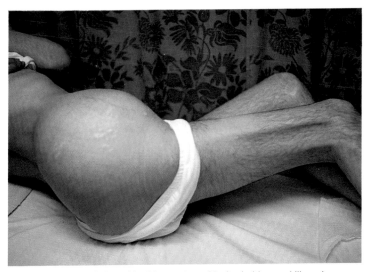

Fig. 226 Extensive soft tissue bleed in a patient with classical haemophilia and pseudotumour appearances.

Treatment
- Prophylactic factor VIII (heat treated) is given before surgery on a regular basis in severe cases.
- Early treatment of bleeds with factor VIII is the mainstay of therapy.
- DDAVP (vasopressin analogue) increases endogenous factor VIII levels and is often sufficient prior to dental procedures.
- Oral antifibrinolytics, e.g. EACA may also be useful to stop minor bleeding.
- If anti-factor VIII antibodies develop, therapy is very difficult. Strategies include high doses of factor VIII, porcine factor VIII and plasmapheresis.
- Social and psychological support.

Von Willebrand's disease

Aetiology
This disease is more common than classical haemophilia. It is an autosomal dominant condition in which there is a deficiency of factor VIII antigen and factor VIII cofactor with variable factor VIII C levels. The factor VIII cofactor deficiency leads to a platelet defect. The severity of the bleeding disorder is very variable.

Investigations
The PTT is prolonged and the PT and TT are normal. Factor VIII C levels may be reduced. The bleeding time is prolonged and there is abnormal platelet aggregation to ristocetin (Fig. 229).

Treatment
DDAVP and EACA are used where possible. If factor VIII replacement therapy is required, fresh plasma may be adequate. Sometimes factor VIII concentrate must be used and the effect is often prolonged. The bleeding time is a good guide to treatment efficacy.

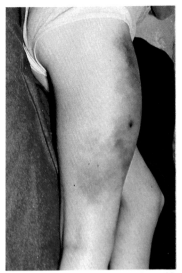

Fig. 227 Soft tissue bleed in a patient with classical haemophilia.

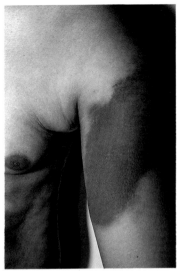

Fig. 228 Result of intramuscular injection in a patient with severe von Willebrand's disease.

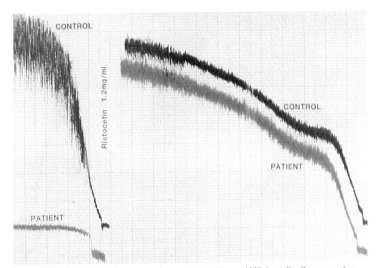

Fig. 229 Platelet aggregation curves in a patient with von Willebrand's disease and a normal control. There is no response in the patient to ristocetin.

30 / **Prethrombotic states**

This refers to any situation in which there is an increased risk of thromboembolism.

Causes
- Circulatory stasis, e.g. immobilization, pelvic tumours, hyperviscosity.
- Increased platelets or platelet aggregability.
- Increased clotting factors.
- Factor V Leiden.
- Deficiencies of coagulation inhibitors:
  —antithrombin III deficiency
  —protein C deficiency (Fig. 230)
  —protein S deficiency.
- Lupus anticoagulant (causes thrombosis and spontaneous abortions—not bleeding; Fig. 231).
- Abnormalities of the fibrinolytic system.

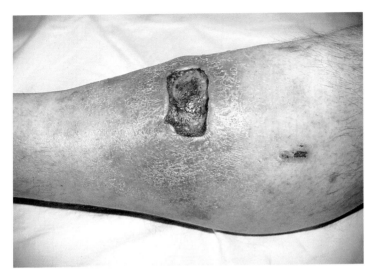

Fig. 230 Necrotic lesion in a case of protein C deficiency on warfarin therapy.

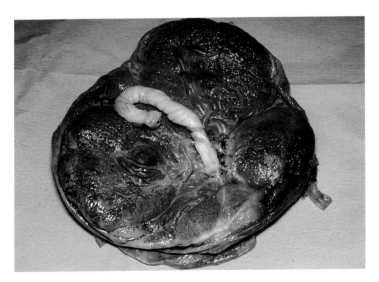

Fig. 231 Infarcted placenta in a case of lupus erythematosus.

31 / **Blood transfusion**

Blood donors   They should be healthy adults under the age of 65 years with no transmissible diseases. Blood is routinely screened for hepatitis B and C, syphilis and HIV.

Blood grouping   Blood for potential donors and recipients is first 'grouped' for the ABO and rhesus systems.

Blood group	Antibodies present	Incidence in UK
A	anti B	36%
B	anti A	14%
AB	nil	3%
O	anti A and anti B	47%
D	nil	85%
d	nil	15%

Subgroups of A occur, 80% being A_1 and 20% A_2. A_2 behaves like a weak form of A_1 and is used in the grouping procedure as a sensitive control.

Although no anti D antibodies naturally occur in d/d patients, immune IgG antibodies readily occur following immunization. Grouping can be done rapidly by looking for agglutination on a slide or tile with the relevant antibodies (Fig. 232). The rapid grouping is usually checked by looking for agglutination in a tube after 90 minutes.

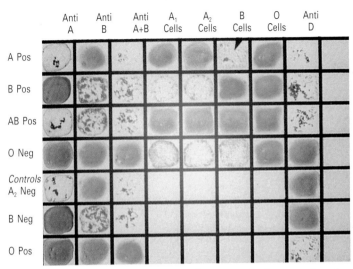

Fig. 232 Tile blood grouping. Agglutination indicates a reaction between cells and serum. Cells or sera from known blood groups are shown down the left. The first three squares and the last square across are the cells reacted against commercial antisera. In between is serum for that individual against known typing cells. Thus serum from an A positive individual reacts with B cells (*arrowed*) but not A_1, A_2, or O cells.

Rhesus grouping is performed by the tube method at 37°C.

Crossmatching Donor cells of the appropriate ABO and Rh groups are chosen and mixed with recipient serum. Incompatibility due to antibodies in the recipient serum is sought by looking for agglutination. This is usually carried out at 37°C in low ionic strength saline and by means of an indirect antiglobulin test with the appropriate controls (Fig. 233). This process is frequently automated.

In many centres, a formal crossmatching is not performed before surgery if the risk of requiring blood is low. In these circumstances the patients' sera is tested against red cell panels to ensure there are no anti-red cell antibodies. Group-compatible blood can then be given after a very rapid crossmatch.

Use of whole blood This should be restricted to cases where both plasma expansion and increased red cells are required. For chronic anaemias, packed cells should be used.

Complications of blood transfusion
- Immediate haemolysis. This usually represents an administrative error in the labelling of the blood or a mistake in the crossmatch (Fig. 234).
- Delayed haemolysis. An antibody not present at the time of transfusion develops rapidly causing haemolysis after 1–2 weeks.
- Febrile and allergic reactions.
- Infections especially hepatitis.
- Heart failure.
- Thrombophlebitis.
- Air embolism with central lines.
- Iron overload in the multiply transfused.
- Massive transfusion may cause potassium and citrate toxicity, acidosis, hypothermia and dilution of platelets and clotting factors.

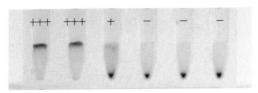

Fig. 233 Bioview crossmatch system. Non antibody-coated red cells spin to the bottom of the bead-filled tube (negative reaction, –). Antibody-coated cells remain at the top of the beads (strong positive, +++) or scattered among the beads (weak positive, +).

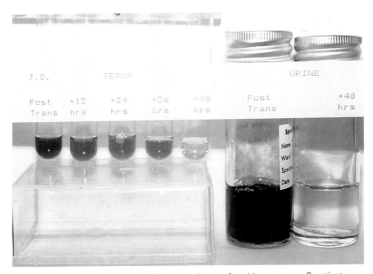

Fig. 234 ABO transfusion reaction. Group A cells transfused into a group O patient resulting in intravascular haemolysis with free haemoglobin in the serum and urine.

Index